Red Moon

Miranda Gray is a professional author and illustrator who has worked on a number of projects in the field of self-help, folklore and spirituality.

Red Moon

Understanding and Using the Gifts of the Menstrual Cycle

MIRANDA GRAY

With best wishes,

Miranda Gray '95

ELEMENT

Shaftesbury, Dorset ● Rockport, Massachusetts
Brisbane, Queensland

© Miranda Gray and Richard Gray 1994

Published in Great Britain in 1994 by
Element Books Limited
Longmead, Shaftesbury, Dorset

Published in the USA in 1994 by
Element, Inc.
42 Broadway, Rockport, MA 01966

Published in Australia in 1994 for
Element Books Limited by
Jacaranda Wiley Limited
33 Park Road, Milton, Brisbane, 4064

Cover illustration by Miranada Gray
Cover design by Max Fairbrother
Design by Roger Lightfoot
Typeset by The Electronic Book Factory Ltd, Fife, Scotland
Printed and bound in Great Britain by
Redwood Books, Trowbridge, Wiltshire

British Library Cataloguing in Publication
data available

Library of Congress Cataloging in Publication
data available

ISBN 1 – 85230 – 496 – 0

Contents

Acknowledgements

My thanks to all those who have helped in the development of this book, either by discussing their own experiences with me or by sharing their own understanding and insights. Special thanks to Naomi Ozaniec for her support and encouragement, and to Julia McCutchen for having confidence in the concept. Finally, thanks to my husband Richard for his help and for continuing to live with me while I worked all this out!

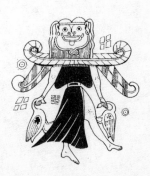

ONE

Introduction

THE AIMS OF THIS BOOK

Modern society's experience of the menstrual cycle is that of a passive event which is acknowledged to happen, but is either ignored or hidden. Women are told that they have to 'cope' with any distresses or needs without bringing attention to themselves, as this is 'part of being a woman'. Because of this, women will often hide their difficulties from others in the fear of being seen as weak or making a fuss about nothing and this lack of communication and social acknowledgement perpetuates the isolation of the menstrual cycle as a hidden and furtive event. *Red Moon* sets out to show that the menstrual cycle is actually a dynamic event which when freed of conditioned and social restrictions can actively affect the physical, emotional, intellectual and spiritual growth of a woman and the society and environment in which she lives.

The menstrual woman lives in a male-orientated society which influences her perception of the world and of herself. This society offers no guidance, structures or concepts for the feelings and experiences of the menstrual cycle, nor any recognition for the expressions which can arise from it. *Red Moon* offers women ways in which they can become more aware of their menstrual cycle and can achieve some understanding of the energies associated with it. Each woman's experience of her cycle is different and the ideas in *Red Moon* are designed to be adapted by the individual reader to suit her own needs.

The approach of *Red Moon* is two-fold. Although it is missing from modern society, a large body of teachings and ideas concerning the menstrual cycle can be found in many legends, myths, folk stories and nursery stories. *Red Moon* offers a reinterpretation of some of these familiar stories and uses the common tales and their inherent symbolism in a new story called *The Awakening* (Chapter 2) as a basis from which the reader may understand the cyclic nature of womanhood. Although concepts and structures are important to aid understanding, they also need to be backed by personal experience and therefore *Red Moon* also suggests ways in which the reader may become more aware of her own cycle, and her perception of it, through her own personal interaction each month.

These two approaches are inter-related. The stories and mythology which contain images relating to the menstrual cycle grew from the personal experiences of women, and so they become a means for the modern woman to gain an understanding of her own experiences of the menstrual cycle. Throughout *Red Moon*, the importance of personal awareness is emphasized with practical suggestions and exercises, some or all of which can be easily incorporated into everyday life. *Red Moon* treats the whole of the cycle as the menstrual experience rather than the time of bleeding alone. The book offers guidance and practical suggestions on methods of interacting with the energies of the menstrual cycle and also considers ways in which women may express their understanding to their daughters and to other women.

THE SOCIAL POSITION OF MENSTRUATION

For centuries, the woman's menstrual cycle has been viewed with something approaching revulsion and contempt; it was seen as dirty a sign of sin and its existence reinforced women's inferior position in male-dominated society. Menstruation is still viewed today as a bio-logical disadvantage to women, making them emotional, unreasoning and unreliable workers.

In the industrialized western culture, which likes to think of itself as 'enlightened', the menstrual cycle is still rarely openly talked about except in medical terms. There are barriers between mothers and daughters, wives and husbands, sisters and friends. Many women go through their lives hating themselves and feeling guilty for being depressed, irritable, bloated and clumsy at certain times in the month. How many women have passed that hatred and fear onto their children, either verbally or in the way they behave? How many women's first period was a frightening experience because they knew nothing about what to expect or at best only the clinical details which did nothing to explain the way they felt? In modern society, where there are no longer any rites of passage, how many girls have actually felt that they had received the gift of womanhood and were given guidance in how to grow with the experience? By learning the gifts of their own menstrual experience and seeing it in a positive light, women will once more be able to guide their girl-children into welcoming womanhood and its cycles.

Many women suffer in their menstruation both mentally and physically and help tends to be available only for fighting the symptoms. The cause, which is obviously being a woman, cannot be helped. The existence of premenstrual syndrome is now beginning to become accepted in modern society, but its effects are still viewed as negative and destructive. Women have had to fight very hard to make society, medical science and the law realize that women pass through an altered state of awareness linked to their menstruation, but there is no longer any structure or tradition which will help women to understand and use that awareness in a positive fashion.

Menstrually active women are cyclic by nature, but with society's linear view of time and events it is often difficult for women to realize this and to acknowledge and make use of it in their lives. Even when women record their monthly dates in a diary, it can be difficult to see them as a cycle of events rather than as a repeating linear pattern. The use of the Moon Dials as a method of recording this information and viewing it in new ways will be considered in Chapter 4. If women become aware that they are cyclic beings during their menstrual lives, then they begin to recognize that they are part of the greater rhythms of the universe and come closer to accepting their true nature and finding harmony in their lives.

The Taboo of Menstruation

The power of menstruation was acknowledged by past cultures and is still acknowledged by a few present-day societies. Those practices which were established by women to help them with the creative energies, however, became largely abused by patriarchal societies which viewed menstrual power as being dangerous to men. Menstruation changed from being sacred and holy to being unclean and polluting. The menstruating woman was seen as a walking source of destructive energy, who held within her femininity a tremendous magical power which could not be contained except by shutting her off from the community and the land itself. This unrestrained magic was felt to contaminate anything with which she came into contact and was particularly dangerous to men, their way of life and their goods and livestock.

At the first sign of bleeding, women were often separated from the community. In many cultures, this meant that the women were confined to a hut, away from the rest of the village, which was shared by all the women of the tribe. The menstruating women were not allowed to touch the implements of daily life and anything which they came into contact with at this time became 'contaminated' and had to be destroyed. In particular, the menstruating women were forbidden to touch anything belonging to a man; it was feared that they possessed the power to cause a man's death or the loss of his hunting prowess. In some cultures, the penalty for women breaking this taboo was death. Other women were allowed to visit menstruating women, but they were forbidden to see or be seen by the men of the village.

Not only was the menstruating woman restricted in where she could go, what she could touch and who she could see, but she was often also restricted in what she could eat. In some cases, she was forbidden to eat meat or drink milk in case she caused the hunting to be bad or the cows to dry up. The menstruating woman was felt to be so unclean that she offended nature, causing the natural order of things to be changed.

The most 'dangerous' time for the community was when a girl-child first started her bleeding. The restrictions placed on the child were often extreme versions of those placed on the adult women. Confinement could last as long as seven years and the girl might be restricted to a small cage, being forbidden to walk on the ground or to see the sun.

Menstrual taboo is not confined just to primitive societies or to the past. In many religions, the menstrual woman is even today restricted both physically and mentally. In Islamic culture a menstruating woman is still refused entry to a mosque; in the past, the penalty for transgression was death. In some Christian cultures, menstruation represents the original sin of Eve, a sin with which every girl-child is born. Christian women are considered never to be free from this sin and have to continually atone for it if they are to enter heaven. This effectively ensures that no woman is sufficiently holy to take an active part in the religion.

Women need to become aware of just how much of their attitude towards menstruation has been shaped by society's history. Once they have realized this, women are enabled to break down this social conditioning and to review their menstruation anew, finding out what it means to each individual, regardless of the view of any other person or group.

THE MENSTRUAL ENERGIES

Within this book, the term 'menstrual' is used to denote matters pertaining to the whole of the monthly cycle, rather than just to the time of bleeding. The creative energies linked to the menstrual cycle have differing orientations and aspects. These menstrual energies are linked to the cycle of the womb. If the egg released at ovulation is fertilized, these energies are expressed in the forming of new life; if it is not fertilized, then the energy is given form in a woman's life in some other way.

The energies of the menstrual cycle must not be restricted or controlled; to block or restrain them can lead them to appear destructive. The energy needs to be accepted as a flow which will express itself in its own way. Fighting this flow can cause both mental and physical pain, because the woman who resists is fighting her own nature and the result can often be aggression, anger and frustration. Menstrual energies find their expression in the many forms of a woman's creative nature.

Withdrawal from society at bleeding was a natural expression of the energies of menstruation. It was a time to teach and to learn and a time to use the collective energies of the whole group of menstruating women. The confinement at puberty was not originally a negative concept but rather one which enabled the wise women to teach young girls the nature of their bodies, of their newly aware energies and of the spiritual traditions which accompanied them. It meant that the post-pubescent woman would emerge in balance and harmony with her nature and be able to use her energies for the community and the land.

TOWARDS AWARENESS

Exercise

It is obviously very difficult in the rush of everyday life to find time to take on one more project. Even finding fifteen minutes to write a diary can be a problem when an extra fifteen minutes in bed can be vital! To understand the energies of your own menstrual cycle and to keep a record of the exercises suggested in the book, you will need to keep some type of diary or journal. To obtain a reasonable representation of your cycle for the Moon Dials, you will need to keep a detailed entry as outlined below for a minimum of three months, although you will begin to have an idea of the form which your cycle takes after the first month.

It is a good idea to continue to jot down any notes, ideas and dreams in a journal after the three months as a way for you to record your insights and experiences. The entries do not need to be lengthy, but do need to include a number of details:

ENTRY

DATE

DAY IN CYCLE

Start the first day of bleeding as number one; if you do not know which day you are on, continue with the rest of the entries until you start your next bleeding.

MOON PHASE

Most of the newspapers will tell you what phase the moon is in; draw a little symbol to show if it is full, dark, waxing or waning.

DREAMS

If you can remember your dreams, write down the basics of the dream or any strong themes or images. You may find that you will remember your dreams initially on waking, but that after a few minutes you will forget them. To try to capture them, either write the dream down as soon as you awake or else mentally replay the dream in detail, impressing on your mind that you want to remember it and then write the dream in your journal when you have time.

FEELINGS

Try to record how you feel during the day. Do you feel happy, low, tired, sociable, withdrawn from the world, intuitive, peaceful? Do you feel drawn to certain activities or styles of clothing? Look at your sexuality; do you feel sensual, loving, giving, spiritual, creative, erotic, wild, demanding, lustful, aggressive, empty? It is not important to note how often you have sex if you have a sexual partner, but try to notice the feelings of sexual energy and the forms they take.

HEALTH

Make a note of any menstrual pains or ailments, any food cravings and whether you feel you are under stress.

It is necessary to become aware of your cycle and the way it affects you, but you also need to look at your menstrual past and to consider the relationships and influences around you then and now. Take time to remember your first bleeding; how much did you know about menstruation at the time? Was it a frightening or embarrassing experience? What was your mother's reaction to it, your family's reaction or those of your school friends or teachers? Also think about how your mother or close female relatives view their own menstruation. What do they call it? Do you have any interaction with them about your menstruation? If you have children how have you or will you teach them about your cycle and if they are girls how will you teach them about their own cycle?

Look at the relationship between your partner, your work colleagues and your friends and menstruation. Is it ignored, treated as 'women's problems', made into a joke or used in a derogatory way? Do you or your partner dislike making love when you are bleeding? Why? Summarize your thoughts in your journal.

The following chapter introduces some concepts and ideas linked to the menstrual cycle taken from different cultures and legends and combined into the single story of *The Awakening*. The themes, imagery and concepts introduced here will be expanded upon in the subsequent chapters.

The purpose of using a story in this way is to encourage you to identify with certain characters and images linked to the menstrual cycle. This identification will bring about the traditional process of initiation, that is, the gaining of knowledge, through the visualization of the imagery in your own mind. Participation with the story, whether through listening or reading, awakens realization and inspiration through the experience of emotions and feelings linking the concepts of the story to the *intuitive* nature of the mind, rather than to the intellect.

The Awakening contains many levels of meaning which you are encouraged to participate in at your own level of understanding. Do not worry if you feel that you do not understand all the meanings in the story, as many of them will become more apparent to you as you work through the awareness exercises later in the book.

After reading and working through the exercises in the book, it is suggested that you return to the story *The Awakening* and its subsequent chapter to compare and reinforce your understanding of your own cycle with the images found in mythology and folk stories.

TWO

The Awakening

Eve lay on her bed in the darkness and sighed deeply. For some reason it had been a really bad day; everything had gone wrong and now she was banished to her bedroom just for fighting with her brother. In angry frustration, she threw her pillow at the door and buried her head in the duvet. From the landing outside her room, she could hear her mother talking and the whining complaints of her brother.

Eve rolled onto her side, her attention drawn by the bright silver light which streamed through the bedroom window. For a moment, it seemed as though time stood still and the murmur of the television and of her family seemed far away. Slowly, Eve climbed off the bed and walked across a room which no longer felt familiar, bathed as it was in the silvery light. At the window, Eve knelt on an old chair piled high with discarded clothes, undid the latch and leaned out into a night which had become warm and magical. A gentle breeze played through the ends of her long hair. Even the city had caught a strange serenity and the noise of the late-night traffic was a low rumble in the background. Her bedroom window faced south and from it Eve had a clear view over the rooftops.

Directly in front of her, in a deepening ultramarine sky, hung the full moon and a single companion star. Silently, Eve made a wish. The moon seemed strange floating above the throbbing city and Eve could feel its magic reaching out to her and gently touching her deepest core. Her body seemed to melt and flow, joining with the moonlight and the earth beneath the house and she knew that above this same place the same moon had shone for millions of years. In sudden realization, time became visible, a shining silver thread which streamed away from Eve into the darkness of the past. With her feet anchored in the earth, Time touched her awareness and a younger city lay before her, alive with fires from the bombs of war. Time touched her again and a small settlement lying between two rivers was attacked by invaders beaching

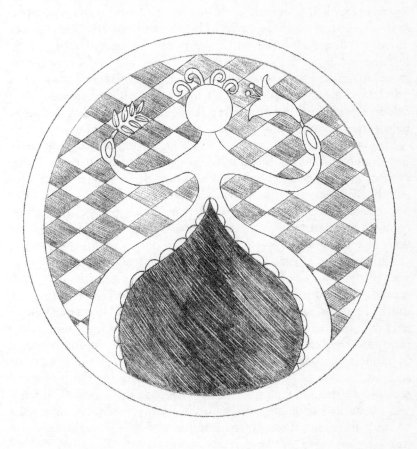

their vessels on the shingle banks. In quick succession the images changed; a small group of people digging a ditch with antler picks; forests displacing the people; and ice in white waves scouring the land clean. Forests, rivers, oceans and deserts advanced and retreated and always the same silver moon shone above. Land rose from the primeval seas and for an instant the small awareness which was still Eve grasped the immense age of the moon and its silent companionship for all that had lived.

From the pivot of creation Time reeled futureward, carrying Eve's awareness with it. Beneath her gaze the first land creatures emerged from the waters of their birth under the full moon's light. In the moonlight a female ape, sitting high in the branches of a tree, reached up her hands to touch the face of the moon and a cavewoman crouching naked and tattooed offered up her newborn child. Eve watched while a priestess clothed in white sprinkled incense on a golden brazier in front of a silver mirror and a small girl with dark hair leaned out of a window and gazed up at the moon.

Still in the haze of silver light, Eve felt the tendrils of Time leave her awareness but the thread of life which linked her with the other moongazers remained. She was kin to all these women, part of a sisterhood which the moon had touched and to which many had responded. Throughout the world, the land, the language, the culture could change but they all watched the same moon, whose light and tides linked them all.

Although the moon's vision had made Eve feel small and insignificant in the passage of time, she now felt part of something special, reaching beyond her everyday life. Eve reached out her hand as if to touch the moon and whispered softly, 'Companion of women, watch over me!' She wasn't sure why she said it, but she felt a strange need to express the sudden bond she felt with the moon. Behind her, as if in a different world, she heard her parents turn off the television set and saw the lights of the house go dark. Although she felt she wanted to stay with the moon all night, sleep tugged at the edges of her mind and she turned reluctantly from the window. Under the duvet, she watched the moon through narrowing eyes until her eyelids grew too heavy to stay open any longer.

Fear pulsed through her sleeping mind. In the darkness, something evil was hunting her. Eve ran blindly through the dark shapes, terror rising, a scream which she was unable to utter forming in her throat. She didn't know what it was that she was running from, she didn't know if it had a form or if it was a ghost or spirit, but she did know that the fear rose from the very depths of her being. Branches and twigs scratched at her face and hands as she fought her way through

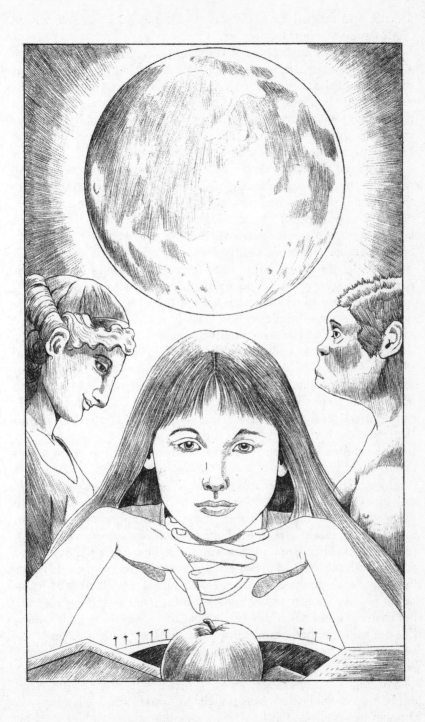

a dense and tangled forest. It was getting nearer; Eve could feel its loathly presence hunting for her.

As she ran, the urgent note of a hunting horn pierced the silent night and for a moment Eve paused, gasping for breath, unsure of which way to run. From the corner of her eye she saw a shadow moving quickly towards her. 'Too late!' her mind cried as she turned and plunged into the grasping undergrowth. Thorns tore at her clothes and legs as she tried to push her way through. In wild panic, Eve looked behind her and felt two more hideous shapes join the first one.

Eve clawed desperately at the bushes; but the more she tried to push through, the tighter the thorns held her. Trapped, her terror broke through and she crouched whimpering, her hands covering her face. Fiercely she prayed that *they* wouldn't find her, but from between her fingers she could see the shadows moving purposefully towards her. She closed her eyes more tightly than ever and sobbed.

Suddenly, a brilliant white light seemed to burst in front of her, burning red against her closed eyelids. Opening her eyes with a start, Eve could just make out the ghosted shape of a woman within the light, facing away from her and towards the shadows. The woman lifted her arms and cried a single command, sending the terrifying shadows slinking and cowering back into the darkness. The woman tilted her head as if listening and Eve could just make out the faint sound of a horn blowing a retreat in the far distance. As she turned towards Eve, the woman's shining aura slowly faded, leaving her standing tall and bright under the silver light of the full moon. With her fear replaced by wonder, Eve cautiously pulled herself away from the thorns and reached out her fingers to touch the Moon Lady's outstretched hand.

The Moon Lady smiled, 'Welcome, child', and it seemed that a million women's voices echoed the words inside Eve's mind. Eve thought that she had never seen such a beautiful woman, her skin a smooth silver-white in the moonlight and her eyes sparkling with its reflection. She wore a long gown of pale blue and a plaid of fabric across her shoulders held in place by an intricate silver brooch. Her hair hung long, pale and free down her back and a simple fillet rested across her brow. Eve felt safe in her presence and a strange feeling stole over her that she had known this lady all her life. The Moon Lady guided Eve out from the dense undergrowth and as they walked through the silver-washed trees the Lady spoke, her voice soft and musical like a bubbling spring.

'This night is very special for you. It marks the turning of the wheel of life from childhood to womanhood. My sisters and I will guide you through this night and although you may not understand all that you will see or feel as you become a woman, you will at least *begin* to understand.

'As a child, your energies are linear; they flow constantly towards the single goal of making you grow both mentally and physically from a baby into an adult. In the change from child into woman, these energies change from linear to cyclic. Your energies will follow a rhythm which will repeat itself about once a month. The colour and taste of your rhythm will be individual to you and I am here to help you to become aware of it, and of the different energies within it.'

Their walk had brought them to a small glade in the forest and as Eve looked up towards the moon she gasped in delight at the myriad diamond stars which danced on the waves of night. For a moment, the sky developed depth and Eve gazed far into the limitless vastness of the universe.

'As a woman, you are linked to the rhythm and beat of the universe both large and small.' The Lady's words fell as a whisper in the vastness of space. 'Back through the generations of time, women have been the link between man and the universe. Through the first menstruation, female apes evolved separately from the rest of the animal kingdom and every bleeding became a clock in tune with the rhythms of the cosmos.'

The words tugged at Eve's soul, making her yearn to leave the restrictions of her body and merge with the turning of the stars. A shiver ran through her spine and, like ripples spreading outward on a pond, the scene wavered and changed.

Eve found herself standing in a huge, dark, circular room, on a floor of black and white tiles. In the centre of the room stood four heavy brass tripods holding bowls of flame and their dim and flickering light surrounded and illuminated a seated figure, her face turned away from Eve. Curiously, Eve walked towards the woman, aware of the Moon Lady following behind her.

On a solidly carved wooden throne sat a woman whose beauty was beyond description. She was dressed in a robe of watery silk and her fine hair hung loose to the floor, where it seemed to grow across and between the tiles. At first she seemed to be covered from head to toe in the finest silvery veil, embroidered with numerous shining jewels, but as Eve drew closer she could see that the gems were in fact tiny spiders, busily spinning the veil. The lady's face was calm and serene and her eyes looked down into a bowl of beaten silver, filled with crystal-clear water which she held on her lap. There was a deep stillness about the lady, as if she herself were timeless. Her hands rested gently on the rim of the bowl and from a cut on the end of one of her fingers a small bead of bright red blood welled. As Eve watched, a drop fell

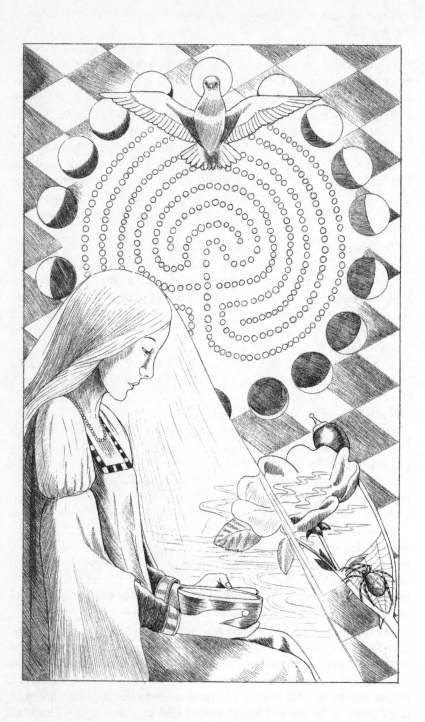

from the lady's hand into the water, which immediately turned red with the blood.

'Who is she?' asked Eve.

'She is the Holder of Measure,' answered the Moon Lady. 'Each drop of blood counts each dark moon and each tear a full moon.'

Under the long eyelashes, a single tear gathered and slowly trickled onto the lady's cheek.

'How long has she been here?'

'Since the first female started to bleed. Throughout time she rests in this place, counting the rhythms of the moon and measuring the cycle of women. Women's time is different from that of men; men follow the sun whilst we follow the patterns of the moon. From women came the first measure of time.'

The Moon Lady reached out and, taking Eve's hand, led her out through an oak door. Outside the door, the forest was lit by a full moon and, turning, Eve saw that she had just left a huge, circular hut with a conical thatch reaching high into the sky like a hill. As the Moon Lady closed the door, she bent down and picked a rose from a bush next to the door frame. She held it out to Eve.

'A gift from the Holder of Measure.'

The rose was pure white in the moonlight, but as Eve held the stem, the centre of the flower deepened to red and the colour spread across the petals to cover the whole flower. Rhythmically, the flower changed red to white to red, the stains washing over the petals in Eve's hands. Eve looked up to question the Moon Lady but as she raised her eyes she noticed that a change had come over the moon. Where before it had been full, now it was waning. As she watched, the moon turned completely dark and then reappeared as a growing crescent. With ever-increasing speed, the moon passed through each of its phases. In her hands, the flower also cycled from white to red; sometimes the white flower matched the full moon and sometimes the red. Watching the patterns, Eve could see that the flower's cycle oscillated around the full and dark moons.

Eve reached out a finger to touch the pulsating flower, but as she did so the white petals suddenly became petal-soft feathers, which launched themselves into the air. Startled, Eve laughed as a pure white dove climbed high into the dark sky.

'Throughout your fertile life your rhythm will be your companion. Sometimes it will be in time with the moon, sometimes longer, sometimes shorter. You will bleed with the full moon and perhaps with the dark moon. All are natural; you are your own rhythm and it is your own cycle which you must learn and accept. All women throughout history are linked together by the rhythms of the moon.'

Eve felt again that sisterhood with the prehistoric women and their link with the moon which she held in her own body.

'Why do you need clocks,' she thought, 'when you are linked to the rhythms and patterns of the earth and the universe?'

A pain in her finger drew her attention back. A thorn from the stem in her hand had pricked her finger and a small bead of bright red blood welled on the tip. The Moon Lady took her hand and carefully wiped the blood away with a white napkin. Taking the thorny rose stem, she wrapped it carefully in the bloodied napkin. Kissing Eve lightly on the cheek, the Moon Lady smiled.

'You have more of my sisters to meet, but first you must rest.'

Eve was about to protest that she was not tired when lethargy washed over her like a flood and she could no longer stop herself from yawning. Still smiling, the Moon Lady led Eve to a mossy patch at the base of a huge oak tree. Curling up between the roots, Eve gave in to the sudden tiredness and allowed her eyes to slowly close, pausing for a second to study the bramble flowers reflecting the moonlight.

Birdsong filled the air. Eve sat up and yawned, feeling refreshed and happy. She leaned against the base of a tall cypress tree, on a rocky hill the colour of golden sand. Around her was a woodland of pines, birches, cypress and olives and in the distance she could just glimpse a small patch of deep blue sea. A hand slipped into hers, pulled Eve to her feet and tugged her into a gentle run. The hand belonged to a young Grecian woman, not much older than Eve, who wore her curling hair bound up on her head with a scarf. Her skin was pure and smooth and her features beautifully shaped. She wore a short tunic of soft material held in place by criss-crossing golden threads across her breasts and soft leather sandals strapped up to her knees. In her other hand she held a small silver bow and across her shoulders was slung a leather quiver.

Finally awake, Eve matched her stride with the girl's and felt the beauty of freedom of movement. As they ran in the sunshine, Eve became aware that they were not unaccompanied. From the corner of her eye, she could make out the running forms of a doe and stag, a hare, a wild goat and a she-bear. Suddenly a lioness broke cover and, matching their pace, ran with them through the woods. In the dappled sunlight, the tawny animal became a streak of liquid light and her eyes burned with golden fire.

Eve felt as though she could run for ever, but finally they emerged from under the trees to stop on the side of a grassy hill which swept down into a dust-coloured plain. Just visible in the heat haze, Eve could see a small bay reflecting the bright sunlight. Tired, but not exhausted, she sat down and stretched out her legs in front of her. The young woman joined her and the lioness settled gracefully at her feet.

'I am Artemis, she of the Shining Bow', the girl said, and tossed her head back. 'I am one of the virgin goddesses.'

Around her neck Eve noticed a small carving of a phallus attached to a leather thong.

'Many things have been written about virgin goddesses and many things have been expected of virginity.' She paused and, leaning over, touched Eve's belly. 'You are a virgin in the modern sense of the word, whereas I am a virgin in the older meaning. I am a woman who looks only to myself; I am self-contained, self-sufficient and self-aware. I celebrate life through my actions; I am complete. I represent the time before the egg is released in the cycle. I am not fertile and given over to the creation of life; I am myself and my energies are mine.'

Artemis touched the phallus around her neck and grinned.

'I am not celibate; I enjoy the sexuality of my body and am complete without the *need* for marriage or a child.'

They stood up and started to walk back towards the trees.

'Every month you will go through a stage of rebirth. After your bleeding you will become virgin-like again. In ancient Greece, there were ceremonies for women to wash their bloodied linen at the end of their moon bleeding and to celebrate rebirth as a complete and whole woman. This is the time to marshal your thoughts, to make clear decisions and to act on them. You are self-confident, self-assured, aware of your body and of its needs. Some men feel threatened by this phase and see these attributes as "masculine", but they are as much a part of being female as being nurturing and caring. They are a gift; use them well.'

Eve felt her belly warm as Artemis spoke and fire raced through her body, making her want to run again. But she paused.

'What happens when your cycle stops when you are older?', she asked.

'Then you become like a virgin again. It is a time for a woman to look at her life, to accept her inner path, if she has not already done so, and walk along it. I am not the one to teach you this yet; there are many other things to learn before you reach that stage of your life.'

They walked for a while in companionable silence but when Eve turned to speak again to the goddess, she found herself alone. She looked around and saw that not only had the goddess vanished, but so had the woods and hillside; she was now standing among the regular lines of a well-tended olive grove. The trees hugged the edge of a cliff and Eve could see the deep Prussian blue of the ocean crashing against the white rocks. Between the trees a woman walked slowly towards her. Eve wondered if this could be another of the Moon Lady's sisters and studied her carefully as she approached.

The woman was tall and elegant, with strong features and piercing, intelligent eyes. Her black hair was pulled back from her face and held in place by gold pins. Unlike the soft fabric of Artemis, this lady wore a layered skirt of white linen and fine gold cloth, stiffened with intricate embroidery and edged with tassles. Across her shoulders she wore a pure white goatskin, held in place by two snakeheaded clasps. On the skin was an embroidered red-gold face with snakes for hair and the edges of the skin were fringed with golden snakes. In her right hand the woman held a long bronzetipped spear and on her feet she wore simple rush sandles.

The heat of the midday sun sent ripples through the air and the shining lady beckoned Eve to the welcome shade of a small olive tree. Beneath the tree was a simple altar and a stone chair. The lady sat and indicated to Eve to sit on the ground at her feet. For a moment the lady's intense gaze held Eve's and then she spoke.

'I am Athene, the Ever-Virgin, the fire which creates the wisdom of women.'

Athene took Eve's hand in one of her own.

'In your cycle, your creative energies are not just for the forming of children, but are also for the birth of idea children.' She touched Eve's forehead. 'You produce the spark of life, you carry it in your body, nurture it and allow it to grow until you bring it out into this world. Children enter this world from the womb, idea children enter through your body, your hands and feet, your voice.' She kissed Eve's hands as though in homage. 'A woman without children is not an incomplete or unnatural woman, her children are the ideas she carries within herself and their birth is the form she gives them in the material world.'

'Where do these idea children come from?' asked Eve, puzzled.

'Your sexuality awakens the energies which sow the seeds of inspiration. The act of sex itself can create both physical and idea children and can be the fire which drives the artist, poet, musician and seer. The art of sex is sacred, it brings the divine into the world.'

Eve felt her fingers begin to feel warm and pulse with the need to create.

'What do these idea children look like?' she asked.

'Idea children can take any form. It does not matter how you express the ideas or what you or other people think of the final child. It is the forming of the child which is important and not the child itself. As with a physical child, your heart is given form and other people's opinions can feel like an attack on your very own soul, but the child must be allowed to grow in its own way in the

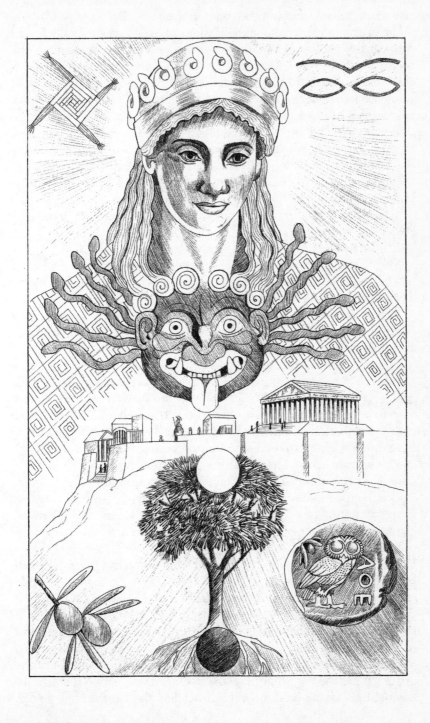

material world. Creating can be a form of meditation or prayer; it is
the act of creation and not the creation itself which reflects the divine.
Women are different from animals; their sexuality is not simply linked
to creating children, but rather its energies are freed throughout the
month in their menstrual cycle. This is the wisdom of women. From
this wisdom comes the ability to make life better, to make implements,
to create structured relationships and communities and the ability to
express the relationship between humanity and nature.'

Athene bent down and picked up a discarded coin lying in the dust
at the base of the altar. She handed it to Eve, who scratched away
the dirt to look at the faces. The coin was small and thick, made of
tarnished silver. On one face was stamped an owl and on the other a
portrait of the goddess wearing a horsetailed helmet.

'The coin symbolizes the energies and the powers I hold,' said
Athene.

Eve looked up from the coin, startled.

'But I thought that money was supposed to be evil and the cause of
all the problems in the world!'

Athene laughed.

'What do you need for a coin to exist?' she asked. 'You need a
craftsperson skilled with their hand and mind to make an object of
such beauty.'

She took the coin from Eve and held it up.

'The coin needs things to buy, so people create from their minds
articles of beauty and practicality. The coin needs to have worth and
so people create a structure for it between themselves. With the coin
comes distribution and trade and where goods and coins meet, markets
develop. From the markets communities grow and cities and kingdoms
evolve with structure, laws, learning and co-operation. The coin is a
symbol of the ability to order life, to create structure and channel
instinct and energies. It is a symbol of civilization.' The coin flashed
in the sunlight. 'The coin is not evil, nor are my energies. Inspiration,
clarity of mind and organization are energies open to all women within
their menstrual cycle.'

The coin flashed once again and this time Eve found herself
looking down on the ancient city of Athens. She saw the ripples
of the goddess's energies in the intricate designs being painted onto
an amphora by a potter, in the skill of a metalsmith working on a
jewelled goblet, in the subtlety of a weaver bargaining with a merchant
on a street corner and in the judgement and counsel being dispensed
in the courtrooms at the seat of government. As Eve looked up, the
image of Athene rose high into the sky, towering above the city. In
her right hand she held a spear, in her left she held a huge golden

shield and a shining golden helmet graced her head. In the setting sunlight Athene's skin turned to radiant light and at her feet a small dark green olive tree grew out of the barren white rock on which she stood. The goddess turned her gaze on Eve, who stood transfixed under the owl-like eyes, and, leaning back, tensed her powerful arms and threw her spear with massive force. A blazing comet of fire streaked across the sky towards Eve.

Eve felt the roaring light overtake her, spinning images from the air around her. In the light, she saw the first communities rise from the dust to bud and blossom and the universe reflected in the first artforms. The light flickered and she saw the structure of society, the warp and weft of the laws, the teachings, judgements and arts. The city pulsed with fire, alive to the energy of the goddess. White and pure, Eve felt the presence of the energy emerging from the darkness within herself. Trustingly, she laid aside her doubt and fear and opened herself fully to the power. For a moment she felt suspended in time and then the world returned in a barrage of sharpened detail and brilliant colour. Every shape, texture, sound and form sent waves of ideas, connections and patterns tumbling through her mind, avalanching until they fell from her lips in a rush of poetry and oracle. As suddenly as it had appeared, the avalanche ceased and, with the fire spent, Eve fell empty to the ground, tired but at peace before the quivering spear transfixing the earth before her.

After a few minutes of rest, Eve rose slowly to her feet but as she reached forward to take hold of the spear, both she and Athene's weapon were snatched by a powerful arm and hauled bodily into the back of a speeding wicker chariot. Bright, ruddy waistlength hair streamed out behind the driver as she urged her two horses faster. In fear and sheer delight, Eve gasped at the skill and strength of the woman, who stood tall and proud, balancing easily against the careering of the chariot. She wore a tunic made from a weave of many colours and a great clasp held a wildly-flapping cloak about her shoulders. Around her neck rested a huge torc of twisted gold thread which shone in the sunlight. Her skin was bronzed and her eyes flashed with fire. The hands which held the reins with measured strength were rough and weatherworn. Beneath the horses' hooves the landscape flashed by; one minute they sped across brown plains, the next through the dappled greens of an oak forest. The speed tore at Eve's hair, forcing the air from her throat in a cry of exultation. She felt stronger than she ever had before, her mind sharp and bright, and the strength which ran through her made her feel able to achieve anything. She was free, independent, a lioness with the strength to fight and to protect.

Just as Eve felt that she would burst with excitement, the woman slowed the horses to a gentle walk through the shade of a forest. Around them was a sense of cool green calmness, but exhilaration still sang in Eve's blood and, laughing, the woman lifted her down onto the grass.

'My name is Boudicca. I am the Queen of the Iceni,' she said, her voice deep and powerful. 'I fight to protect and serve, never to destroy. I am true Victory, the arbiter of peace. I am committed to others and to causes, and I sustain that commitment.'

The Queen descended from the chariot and strode towards one of her horses. Checking its harness, she said, 'In Celtic times a woman was respected. She held land and power in her own right and was respected for her judgement and the qualities she brought to the community. It was the women who goaded their warriors into action, but it was also the women who arbitrated for peace. They were the force behind the tribe and their men.'

She stroked the horse's neck in affection.

'You are experiencing the strength of womanhood, the radiating dynamism of the light phases, but later you will experience the loss of that energy as it is transformed into darkness. Do not look behind you and long for the light or you will miss the gifts of the darkness. Look within the darkness, accept its powers and see the light awakening out of it.'

The Queen turned and leaped into the chariot with the grace of a deer. She lifted her arm in farewell and, slapping the reins against the horses' backs, she commanded them forward.

The chariot sped across the forest in a flash of sunlight until it became a point of light in the distance. Eve, waving frantically, saw the small silhouetted figure of the Queen turn and wave before she disappeared carrying the daylight with her. Eve was left with her arms in the air and a cry on her lips. As she lowered her arms slowly, a slight sadness crept into her mind; she had liked Boudicca.

Once again Eve stood in the moonlit forest and standing quietly next to her was the Moon Lady. They walked together through the forest in silence until the energy of the Queen's ride had transformed itself within Eve into a feeling of calm assurance and harmony.

The Moon Lady brought them out into a clearing, at the centre of which stood a beautiful tree with a silvery-pink trunk. The trunk divided into two outstretched branches containing a bounty of red fruits and the full moon seemed to sit in the upper branches, its light reflecting in the pool of dark blue water surrounding the small island on which the tree grew. Twisting roots hung from the soil into the waters of the pool.

'This is your Womb Tree,' said the Moon Lady and she touched Eve's belly just below her navel. In answer to her touch, Eve felt a warmth grow around the presence of her womb lying within her body. In front of them, the Womb Tree responded, glowing with energy.

'The pool of water is your subconscious mind and the roots of the Womb Tree reach far down into its depths. Your mind and your womb are linked; what happens in your womb is reflected in your mind and what happens in your mind is reflected in your womb.'

Eve felt at peace and in harmony with the tree and felt drawn towards it. She walked to the water's edge and looked into the branches, longing to touch them. The leaves of the tree, reaching across the pool, rustled and whispered her name.

'Eve, Eve!' they sang, 'Take a fruit from your tree.'

As she reached up to a branch which hung low over the water, she gasped and quickly drew her hand back. Amongst the leaves and fruit coiled a small golden-green snake. It lifted its triangular head and hissed.

'I am the guardian of the tree.' Its small jewelled eyes glinted in the moonlight. 'If you take this fruit, you will become a woman and will inherit all the powers which womanhood brings. You will bleed with the moon; you will become cyclic, never constant, always changing with the phases of the moon. Within your body will awaken the powers of creation and destruction and in your intuition you will hold knowledge of the inner mysteries. Your life will become a path between two worlds, the inner and the outer, with the demands each will make on you. All the gifts of womanhood have to be accepted and cherished; if not, the gift can destroy you.' The snake uncurled. 'The gift is not an easy one to accept; how much easier it would be to remain a child.'

Eve paused and then, on impulse, reached up and plucked a fruit. As she did so, the serpent swiftly struck her and before she could react, surged down her body and into her belly. She felt a warmth between her legs and suddenly a rainbow of vibrant energies spilled like water from her vagina. They poured from her body, touching her head, her throat, her hands and feet. In her mind she heard a single note resonate up through her feet and fill her whole body with sound. She felt the energy expand outwards from her, touching everything, making her at one with creation. Poised, she became the pivot between the energy and the world around her. She raised her arms above her head and screamed in sheer delight, releasing the energy into the world, sending it spiralling upward in the form of sound. With immense calm, she felt the energy lying dormant within her and realized her own ability to

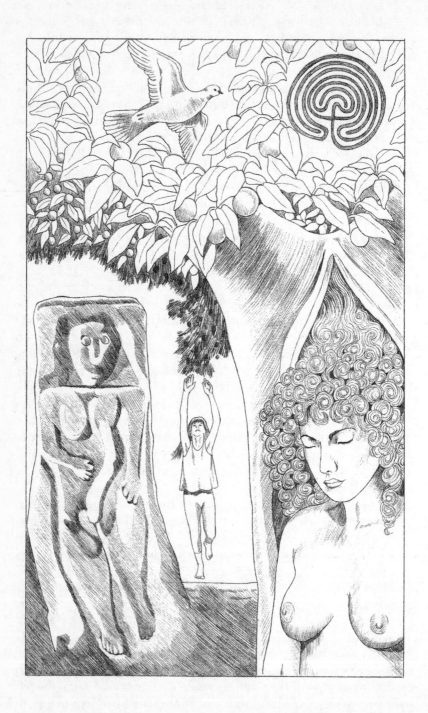

raise it again at will. Looking down, she saw within herself the snake lying coiled under her belly.

She turned to leave the tree and found the Moon Lady standing beside her.

'You have now taken on the powers of womanhood. As you grow more experienced in your cycle, you will need to find how best to use those energies in your life. But you are not alone in this search; there are those within who will guide and support you throughout your menstrual life. There are many more things my sisters and I will show you this night which will help you to use your gift. Touch your tree once more.'

Eve reached up to the tree and gently touched a twig. As if that touch had unlocked a door, the trunk of the tree split open to reveal a lining of crimson. Inside stood a naked woman, her eyes closed and her curling auburn hair forming capillaries in the tree's lining. Eve felt the tree move within her, to merge with her own womb. In her mind she felt the roots of the tree linking her to her womb and she felt the moon lying in both her mind and her womb's branches. The fruit in her hand gradually faded to nothing, leaving her standing alone in the dark clearing.

A flash of white caught Eve's eye and standing in front of her she noticed a large white hare. The gleam from its coat lit the clearing in a soft silvery glow. Dark eyes full of stars and knowledge stared up at her and Eve noticed a small red-jewelled collar about its neck. In the light from the hare's coat Eve saw that the clearing was no longer empty but was filled with animals of all types, silently watching her. She caught her breath at their beauty and power; each animal radiated grace and intelligence and all were painted white by the soft light. Dark eyes sparkled with humour and Eve felt drawn towards them without fear, as though she had known of them for a very long time. Amongst them she saw a huge and powerful bull, a roughcoated wild horse, a shining silver unicorn, a white dove, a small green snake and a beautiful butterfly. Most of the animals seemed to wear some form of jewellery or carried a gift or an artefact of some kind. Eve knew that if she spoke, they would answer her. The hare loped over and sat down without fear between two lionesses. There was a feeling of love and understanding which bound all the animals to the hare and which reached out to pull Eve also into its net.

'These are the Moon Animals,' said the hare, its voice as soft and silvery as its coat. 'They carry the mysteries of the moon and bring messages from your inner world. They live in your dreams and in the realms of faery where talking beasts lead to magical wonders and sources of ancient wisdom.'

A pure white owl swooped, landing close to Eve in a whisper of air. It turned its face towards her, its eyes holding the knowledge of time.

'They offer guidance and counsel, for they hold the instinctual knowledge of your cycle. They bring the grace and harmony which comes from living in tune with your true nature. A Moon Animal may announce your ovulation or bleeding in your dreams or bring dreams whose images can guide you to your cycle and help you to maintain your conscious link with your own rhythm. Remember these dreams and bring them into your waking life. This night especially, remember your dreams, for an animal dreamed of at first blood can have a special relationship with you throughout your life.'

It seemed to Eve as though the hare was smiling as it spoke. The animal turned and then very slowly loped towards Eve carrying something carefully in its mouth. It dropped the gift at Eve's feet and sat back on its haunches. In delight, Eve saw a small white egg wrapped in a bright red ribbon. As she picked it up, she felt a great love within herself which made her want to care for all those around her. A sigh ran through the animals.

'This is your first egg,' said the hare, 'your time of ovulation. The strengths and energies which you felt as a virgin have matured into those of the mother. Do not waste these energies; in the past, women were acknowledged as being strong and dynamic, as well as having the strength to care and nurture. At ovulation the energies are different; they deepen to an expression beyond yourself. You become aware of the deeper level of yourself and of an ability to love and care without sense of self. At this time your creative desire reflects the world around you.'

Eve felt the calmness of the clearing wash over her and became aware of the full moon shining both in her mind and womb, but also in the night sky. She felt in harmony with the moon and all around her and experienced a sense of strength enabling her to give to others in the knowledge that she could nourish and sustain them. The full expression of her soul seemed to shine through her heart, eyes and hands.

'In this time of light you may dream of eggs or of Moon Animals. Remember these dreams and recognize them as announcing your ovulation.'

The hare turned and hopped a little way before pausing as though in invitation for Eve to follow. After a moment's hesitation, Eve followed the hare and the Moon Animals faded from her sight as darkness returned to the clearing.

The hare led Eve through the forest into a meadow full of sunlight.

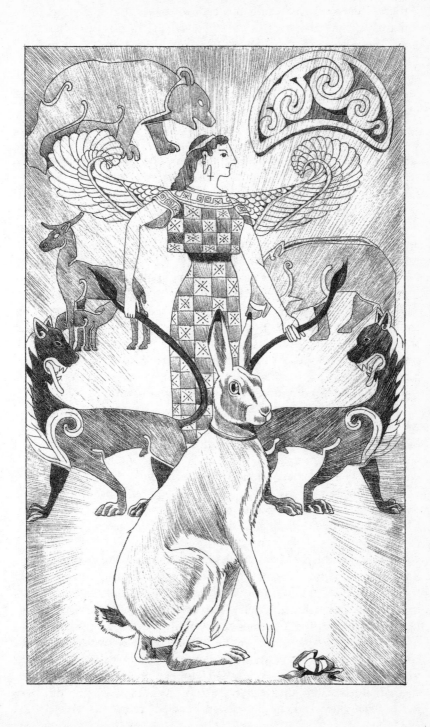

Around her hung the scent of meadow flowers and everything was
vibrant with the energy of life. As Eve walked through the knee-high
grass, she noticed that the flowers teemed with bees and other insects.
Large oxeye daisies turned their heads towards the sun and wild poppies
splashed the meadow with brilliant red. Eve stopped walking and
breathed in the elixir of life surrounding her, wanting to stay and
enjoy the beauty.

Impatiently, the hare urged Eve onwards towards a grassy mound
in the centre of the meadow. At the base of the mound, a series of
white stone steps led down into the earth. The hare stopped with its
front paws resting on the top step. For some reason, Eve felt uneasy;
nevertheless, she started downwards nervously.

At the bottom of thirteen steps, Eve found a carved archway lit by
a single rush torch held in a wall bracket. Across the archway hung
a beautiful green curtain, embroidered with all types of animals, birds
and plants. At the apex of the stone arch, amongst intricate carvings
which echoed the curtain's design, was a cuplike socket. Cautiously,
Eve pulled the curtain aside and entered a shadowy domed room.
The room was completely circular, with a red carpet running across
the stone floor from Eve to a dais on the other side of the space. In
the centre of the dais was a stone throne with a deep red cushion and
on either side of the platform stood two other archways hung with
plain red and black curtains. As Eve watched, one of these curtains
was pulled aside and another lady entered the room.

She was tall, dark haired and dark eyed and although her features
were quite angular, her mouth was full and sensual. She wore a gown of
brilliant scarlet which was cut low and fitted tightly across her breasts
and hips, flowing in great folds to the floor. Around her waist hung a
girdle of gold embroidery and as she walked across the room her body
swayed rhythmically from side to side. There was an aura of power
about her, of sexuality, of hunger and of darkness. Her eyes flashed
with promise. Eve felt uncomfortable, both frightened and fascinated
by the woman.

'Come!' said the Red Lady curtly, her voice sharp and commanding.
She walked to the archway from which she had just entered, held
back the curtain and gestured Eve to go through. Inside was darkness.
Entering and then turning quickly around, Eve could see no trace of
light from beyond the curtained doorway. Her initial fear was quickly
overtaken by tiredness and lethargy; the darkness was warm and
comforting and Eve felt no desire to move or to do anything. She began
to feel irritated that the Red Lady had left her alone in the darkness and
this initial irritation quickly grew into annoyance and frustration. Eve
felt her face flush and the muscles in her body tense.

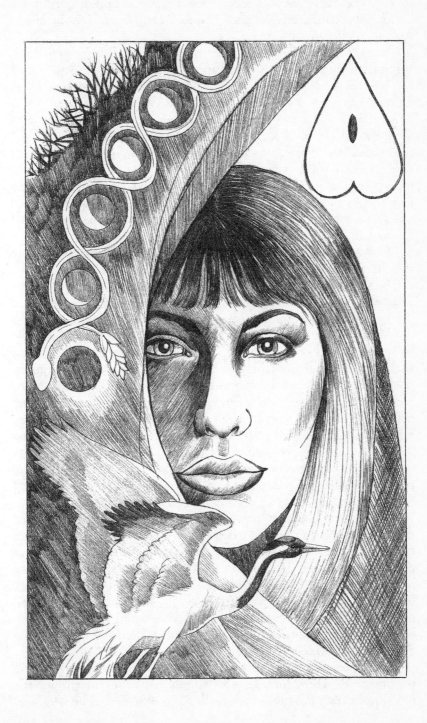

Very gradually, the area around Eve began to lighten, until it was bathed in a harsh, bright light. The Red Lady stood in front of Eve holding a full length mirror.

'Where have you been? I've been waiting for you!' snapped Eve and instantly regretted being so rude and aggressive.

The Red Lady met Eve's gaze and held it for what seemed an eternity.

'Look,' she said and pointed to the mirror. Eve stepped forward for a closer look and found a naked reflection of herself. Puzzled, she studied the image carefully, for although the image was without doubt herself, there was something wrong. Her hair was lank and greasy, her face spotty and her breasts and belly were swollen and painful. As she looked, Eve began to feel dizzy; her head ached and she felt so miserable that tears cascaded down her cheeks and she hid her face in her hands.

'What's happened to me?' she cried. 'I look horrible. I hate myself!'

The voice of the Red Lady cut through her self-pity.

'Look again,' she said sharply, 'this time with your inner self!'

The light had softened and Eve tentatively raised her head. In the dim light she saw her breasts shining and round like full moons. Her belly was domed like the hills of the earth, making her body feel sensual with the curves of womanhood. She felt her body with her hands, not rejecting it but awakening to the change in it. She remembered pictures she had seen of ancient goddesses, full breasted and round bellied, and felt an acceptance of this shape wash over her. In the mirror her hair gleamed with health and her skin became luminous.

'Look at your womb,' said the Red Lady softly.

In the mirror Eve could see her own Womb Tree in her belly. The tree was swollen and red, pulsing with energy in a globe of water. Eve felt the energy pulling her inwards and suddenly she fell with it.

Around her, darkness flowed like water, as though she glided downwards through the murky depths of a lake. Above her green light diffused through the darkness and below her was the deep red-black of primal ooze. She fell slowly into the ooze until its red darkness covered her head. A single breath of the darkness sent power surging through her body, forcing Eve to dance, and as she moved eddies of red and black stirred around her. Eve felt the darkness within as though she were submerged in chaos and in the primal matter from which all life is born and to which all life returns.

In the murk she saw a glint of light and a crescent moon piercing the gloom. Reaching for it, Eve found that what she thought was the moon was in fact the horns on a bull's skull, bleached white with age.

Holding the horns like a dagger, Eve whirled around and around in the darkness, moving to her own rhythm, reaching for her own crescendo of movement. Energy spun around her and in total exuberance she could see lines of power twisting out of her womb and coiling off into the darkness like red snakes. Tipping her head back, her hair flying, she shrieked with delight. The power was raw and savage, she was the Destroyer, the Devourer. A necklace of skulls swung from her shoulders and a girdle of severed arms from her waist. In her dance she cut away the old, mercilessly forcing change and the continuance of time.

Suddenly, booming through the fluid like a drum, a single word commanded: 'Rise!'. With unexpected and unaccustomed grace, Eve pushed upwards through the gloom towards the green shadows above. Breaking the surface of the water, Eve emerged into a huge black cavern. In the centre, towering above her, was an enormous statue of a goddess roughly carved from black granite and burnished until it shone. The goddess stood with her hips buried in the floor of the cavern and her arms reaching out, one downwards towards Eve and one reaching high into the upper darkness. Eve climbed out of the pool and took a few steps towards the image. From below, she could see that the statue's eyes were closed and a single black gem graced its brow.

'Weave!' The word echoed through the rocks and into Eve's body. Suddenly the gem on the goddess's brow blazed with light and threads of stars sprang from the statue's fingertips. All things were touched by these threads, which connected and reconnected all around and through Eve, tying her into the pattern. Beneath her feet the pulse of power from the pool throbbed. Caught between the two streams of energy, Eve raised her arms and let the fire loose from her fingers. No longer restrained, the energy rushed forward, finding form in a thread of stars which Eve wove about her. At one with the goddess, she directed the energy into creation, her conscious mind guiding the flow but not controlling the shape or form. Eve realized that the power to destroy and create were the same force and she knew that she had the ability for both within her. With her new clarity of sight, she could see how everything in the universe was connected and knew that by guiding her power into the material world she could weave her threads into prophecy, magic, art and love. With the energies balanced, Eve stood in wonder, gazing up at the galaxies and stars which shone in the roof of the cavern.

A doorway opened in the cavern wall and a dark figure silhouetted against the light beckoned her. As Eve crossed the cavern floor, she walked with the grace and poise of one who knows herself, who has accepted herself and who has the ability to take responsibility for her

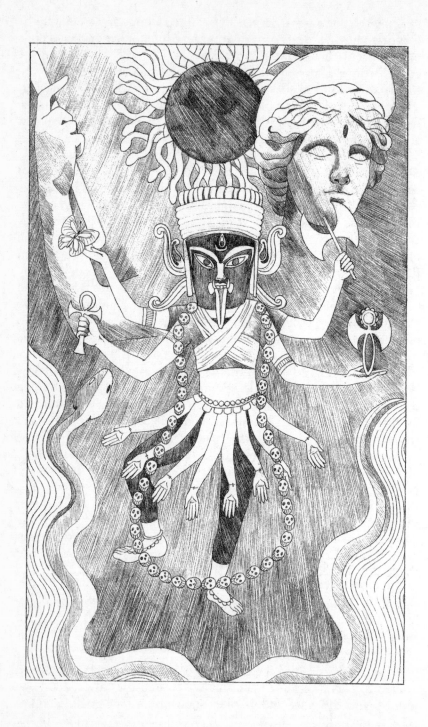

power. Eve strode confidently, aware of the hidden side of life in the world around her.

Walking through the curtained doorway, Eve discovered a long wooden hall lit by a bright central fire. Behind the fire, sitting on a wooden throne, sat a woman covered from head to foot by a translucent red veil. Through the fabric, Eve could just make out the outline of her features. She had long black hair tied into large plaits each weighted with a small golden apple, her skin was porcelain white and her lips a deep shade of red. The shadow of her hands folded in her lap showed them to be long and delicate.

'Welcome, Walker between the Worlds,' said the Lady. It seemed to Eve that she heard the rustle of autumn leaves in the voice.

'I am Sovereignty.' The Lady lifted her arms beneath the veil in welcome.

'I see that you carry the glow of the red veil. Welcome, daughter-priestess.' Eve felt that there was something magical about the Lady and that she should be in a castle of shining towers rather than an empty wooden hall.

'See about you my land.' Eve stretched out her awareness and saw the land lying within the hall. Lines of light reached out from each point, criss-crossing the landscape. Eve took a step forward and noticed that her movements rustled the fabric of the white robe which had become her garb. As she walked towards the fire, each swing of her hips changed the patterns of the lines around her. The season of the landscape changed and she could smell the scents of winter. From the winter darkness she saw the light of spring emerge and felt the seasons flow rhythmically through her body.

Eve reached down into herself to the core of her creative energies and willed them to rise through her body. As the energy reached her fingers she held it there in control, aware of the cycles within her body and the land, ready to weave patterns in both of the worlds around her. The Lady stood up and walked towards Eve, the lines of the land emanating from her body and spiralling back to meet her. All the other women and goddesses whom she had met had been taller than Eve, but Eve quickly became aware that this Lady was about her own size. Although slight, the Lady held a majesty about her which made Eve think of her as a faery queen. In the Lady's hands was a girdle of the finest green silk, richly embroidered with silver pomegranates and golden corn, which she fastened about Eve's hips.

'You are now my representative,' she said. 'You have the power to see both worlds, the inner and the outer. You have the magic to create patterns and ripples in the fabric of both of these worlds. You can touch the web of prophecy, of initiation and of life itself. This is your gift of moon bleeding. You know instinctively of both worlds and at the time of darkness you can walk between these worlds and mediate their energies.

'The modern woman walks in the world of science and technology as well as the world of nature and intuition. These worlds are not absolutes, but rather they mesh together. Both worlds are equally real to a woman and she has the ability to balance them in a flow of awareness from one to the other. It is by this ability that all women are wise women, all women are priestesses.

'A woman who is aware of her cycle must be true to it, but she is also responsible for the use of her energies, their expressions and their effects on others. Responsibility does not mean that she should not use her abilities, but that she should not hide behind her menstrual cycle or use it as an excuse. The responsibility which comes with the gift is great; it is to yourself, to other women, to the community, the land and to future generations.'

Sovereignty raised her hands in blessing.

'Dance your patterns, weave your spells, write your poems, sing your stories, paint your beauty, give birth to your children.'

Eve felt overwhelmed with love for the Lady and for the land and tears fell from her eyes. As each sparkling droplet fell onto the ground, a single white flower formed.

The scene of the land and the hall gradually dimmed, leaving Eve once again in darkness. Abruptly, the curtain was pulled aside once again and Eve saw the Red Lady standing in the doorway to the domed room. When she walked through, Eve found herself on the opposite side of the dais to the one she had entered. Looking at the Red Lady, Eve no longer felt threatened by her sensuousness or the hidden darkness in her eyes. The Lady smiled at Eve's recognition.

'You have accepted what you are but now you need to be true to your nature and this is not always easy. The darkening moon is a time to reserve your physical energies, but it is also a time of great sexual and creative energies. You may find yourself speaking your mind, unable to accept the mundane or routine with the tolerance which you have for the rest of the month. This is the gift of truth, but it may arise out of anger and frustration, from being denied the chance to be true to your nature at this time. From this anger, the energies can become destructive; they can bring pain to yourself and to others, rather than being channelled and guided to constructive and creative use.

'The destructive nature of women was recognized in past times, but was accepted as a part of her creative nature. The woman gives, but she also takes. She is the line of continuity, but she is also broken into cycles. She creates the new, but also destroys the old. Use your destructive energies with wisdom and never forget that destruction and creation are not separate. Being aware of your cycle and the nature of your energies, you carry the responsibility for your actions. It is easier to blame the body and to separate the mind from it than to work within the rhythm and to change your life accordingly.'

The Red Lady climbed the three steps to the top of the dais.

'You are woman. You are strong because you are not constant, because the rhythm of change is the rhythm of the universe.'

As the Red Lady sat on the stone seat, her image changed; the skin paled, the hair lightened, the features softened and the red dress turned to moonwashed blue. With little surprise, Eve recognized the familiar figure of the Moon Lady.

'Yes,' said the Moon Lady in reply to Eve's unspoken question, 'we are the same, but at different times. During the month I am part Moon Lady, part Red Lady but only at the turning points of menstruation and ovulation am I wholly one or the other.'

She stood up, walked down the steps and indicated for Eve to sit on the throne.

'Do not be afraid,' she reassured.

Tentatively, Eve mounted the steps and sat on the red cushion. Still tense despite her increased awareness and understanding, she sat straight and erect, her eyes searching those of the Moon Lady. Gradually, she became aware of a change in the pure white robe around her body. As Eve watched, the hem of the robe turned a delicate pink, then a rich ruby red, the crimson hue spreading upwards to cover the whole garment. Within seconds, Eve was clothed entirely in a robe of blood red. With a sudden feeling of detachment, Eve drew her awareness away from the room and her immediate surroundings. Deep within the welcoming darkness, she became aware of the spiderweb of threads which linked her to the great black goddess. In the depths of herself, Eve thought that she could hear her voice:

'I am the invisible in all things. I am the potential, the darkness of the womb before rebirth.'

When her awareness of the world around her returned, the Moon Lady was standing next to her. The need to stay and the desire not to move were strong. The Moon Lady helped Eve to her feet, but it was the Red Lady who accompanied her down the steps to a small alcove in the wall. Eve climbed up onto a small shelf covered with soft, thick furs and lay quietly in the fading light, feeling the ability for speech or further thought slipping away from her. The Red Lady covered her with a skin.

'Sleep the rest of this night here in the protection of the earth's belly. Remember your dreams and don't forget those that you have met.'

She bent over, kissed Eve and stood watching as Eve's eyes closed and the scene dissolved into darkness. In the warmth of sleep Eve smiled as she heard a fading voice call: 'Remember, remember'.

Sunlight streaming through her bedroom window fell on Eve's face and kissed her gently awake. She felt relaxed and peaceful and lay quietly under the duvet, wishing that she could stay there all day. From somewhere inside her, the night's dreams blossomed into Eve's waking mind. In the light of day, the people and places which Eve had visited, which had seemed so intense and real, were blurred and far away yet Eve was left with a sense of peace and understanding, and with the notion of a promise soon to be fulfilled.

The familiar noises of the rest of the family rising stirred Eve, and yawning and stretching she sat up in bed. As she moved her body, she felt an uncontrollable warm trickle between her legs. Quickly grabbing a handful of tissues from the bedside table, she dabbed at the damp and brought the tissues up to find them covered in the bright red stain of fresh blood. At that exact moment, her mother walked into the room and saw the bloody tissues in Eve's hand. Eve quickly explained to her anxious mother where the blood had come from. With a glint of amusement in her eyes, Eve's mother disappeared for a few moments and returned carrying a handful of pads, handing them to an enquiring Eve.

'I knew it was due soon,' she said, by way of explanation. She smiled and sat next to Eve on the edge of the bed. She pulled Eve to her and lovingly hugged her with tears in her eyes. 'My child is becoming a woman,' she whispered.

THREE

The Dark of the Moon

The use of storytelling and fable as a framework with which to give guidance, understanding and realization is a very ancient tradition in most societies. Many cultures held their storytellers in great respect, because they controlled the power of myth; that is, the ability to open up the intuitive awareness of the inner truths within the listener and to enable them to identify with the rhythms and energies of the universe.

Until fairly recently, only the wealthy and higher classes of society had access to education and were able to read and write, and in many parts of the world this is still the case. Within many of these oral societies, knowledge, wisdom and learning were passed on between tribes and between generations in the form of stories which taught the community about the structure of the universe, the nature of its energies, the gods and goddesses who influenced the lives of the people, the rhythms of the land and the place of humankind within it. The storytellers spoke in images and symbols which rose in the listener's mind during the telling and stayed in the subconscious, where they became integrated with everyday awareness.

Within the stories, a common device was the use of the *archetype* or representative character; these are universal images which reflect certain truths to which people respond on an inner level. Even today, the modern storytelling media use archetypes in films, books and plays, for both adults and children. Horror movies depict the sexual woman linked with death, or the frightening old crone; adventure films depict the helpless virgin who needs to be rescued and inevitably falls in love with her rescuer; and the foundation of family life is depicted as the 'good mother'. The archetype is often carried beyond the screen role in the myth and image which is carefully constructed around the actress herself as 'screen goddess' or 'sex siren'.

For earlier societies, the archetype represented a learning device.

Through identification with the image, the listener would undergo an inner realization, whether consciously or subconsciously, and through that realization could awaken and express the energies of the archetype.

One of the most common archetypes which appeared within many cultures is that of the universal feminine force, the 'Great Goddess'. Often, this image was depicted as three separate female figures or goddesses, representing the life cycle of all women: the Maiden, the Mother and the Crone or old woman.

The Maiden was generally portrayed as energizing and dynamic, reflecting the increasing light of the waxing moon, and was associated with the colour white. The Bright Mother was portrayed as nurturing and fertile, reflecting the radiating light of the full moon, and was associated with the colour red. The Crone was portrayed as the holder of wisdom, the gateway to death and the path to the powers of the inner world. She reflected the increasing darkness of the waning moon which leads to the hidden aspect of the dark moon and was associated with the colours blue or black.

The term 'crone' was used to describe a woman whose menstrual cycles had ended and it was generally believed that women in this phase of life absorbed their menstrual blood each month, thus opening up and making available its powers of creativity, magic and insight. In many societies, a post-menstrual woman was regarded as a 'wise woman' or enchantress whose ability to prophesy and commune with the spirits was greatly respected. The modern image of the crone has lost its power and older women are treated with little respect, almost regarded as surplus to society's requirements.

The description of the life cycle of women is, however, incomplete without a fourth phase, the hidden aspect of the goddess, generally depicted separately from the light triplet. This was the dark mother or terrible mother. She was portrayed as death and as the soul of the divine to which all returned to be reborn. In the life cycle of a woman, this phase represented the soul released at death.

The different aspects of a woman's whole life could thus be segmented and represented by different aspects and archetypes of the divine. However, the lunar cycle was also recognized as an expression of the divine feminine with the land and within women, and many archetypal figures can also be found in mythology and folklore which represent different aspects of the mentrual woman. The young beautiful *Virgin* or innocent maiden represented the pre-ovulatory phase of the waxing crescent moon, the dynamic energies of spring, and the energies of renewal and inspiration. The good *Mother* or Queen represented the time of ovulation, the full moon and the fullness of the energies of Summer. She held the energies of fecundity, sustenance and empowerment. The pre-menstrual *Enchantress* or witch represented the withdrawing energies of Autumn and the increasing darkness of the waning moon. She was a sexually-powerful woman who had the power of magic and the ability to enchant and challenge men; she was either beautiful or ugly, and was generally portrayed in stories as having the ability and power to use her body and her sexuality as part of her enchantment. The Enchantress represented withdrawal and destruction, and often appeared as the initiator of death or disaster necessary for growth. Finally, the ugly old woman or hideous *Hag* represented the menstrual phase of the withdrawn energies and lost beauty of the land in winter. She was the dark moon, and pregnant with the energies of transformation, gestation and inner darkness.

These four images of *virgin, mother, enchantress* and *hag* appear throughout folklore and legend, linking the cycle of the seasons not only to the cycle of the moon but also to the monthly cycle of women. Interpretation of the female mysteries from a modern perspective almost always omits the significance and experience of the menstrual cycle. The mythologies originally expressed not only the external rhythms and energies of life, but also the internal rhythms and energies experienced by menstrual women. These rhythms were so intricately linked with women's own fundamental understanding of the moon, the land and the goddess of life that the modern oversight – due largely to cultural taboos – would have been unthinkable to women in the past. The archetypes of the Virgin, Mother, Enchantress and Hag each offer understanding of the true nature of women and underline the need for women to become aware of this nature.

The stories which reveal this knowledge of the feminine are not just those which are obviously linked to ancient religions but they are also those handed down as stories for children. These so-called 'nursery' stories hold a wealth of ancient symbolism and wisdom originating from early oral society.

We now examine in more detail some of the images and archetypes which appear in 'The Awakening' and their traditional roots and origins.

THE DUAL FEMALE

In many stories, women are depicted as a duality; they are either considered in a positive aspect as a chaste virgin or good mother or in a negative aspect as a destroying, ugly witch or evil, beautiful enchantress. The original meaning of the story is often distorted beyond recognition by the influence of the woman's role as perceived by a dominating male society. The darker aspect of women is portrayed as destructive, but it is in many cases the initiator to a new stage of life or awareness. This can be seen in the stories of *The Loathly Lady* from Arthurian legend and in Grimm's *Snow White* and *Sleeping Beauty*. These stories can in fact be considered as *menstrual myths*; that is, teachings relating to the experiences of the menstrual cycle and the transition of a girl into womanhood.

The story of *The Loathly Lady* begins when King Arthur is challenged and beaten by a mysterious dark knight. Instead of killing Arthur, the knight sets a riddle which must be answered within three days otherwise Arthur will forfeit his life and his land. The riddle is: 'What is it that a woman most desires?' On his return to Camelot, Arthur stops every available woman and asks the question; unfortunately he receives as many different answers as the number of women he asks! Finally, Arthur comes across a hideously deformed and ugly old woman sitting in the woods who claims that she can answer the riddle, but will do so only if Arthur grants her a wish. In desperation, Arthur agrees to the bargain and is told the answer to the riddle, saving his life and kingdom. However, he is horrified to discover that the price which the hag demands is to marry one of Arthur's knights.

Introducing the Loathly Lady to his court, Arthur is not surprised to find that she is met with horror and repugnance by each of his knights and the thought of marriage to such a hideous bride is too much for almost all of them. However, the gallant Sir Gawain finally volunteers for the task and to the amazement of the court he marries her amid much ceremony.

On their wedding night, when Gawain takes the hideous old woman to bed, she is suddenly transformed into a young and beautiful lady. She explains that she is under an enchantment and that by marrying her Gawain has already released half of the spell, but that if he can answer a question correctly, he can free her from the spell completely. The lady then asks the question: 'Would you rather have me beautiful by day or by night?' Gawain is unable to make a decision; if she is beautiful by night, she will be an acceptable and desirable lover, but if she is beautiful by day, he will win envy and status within the court. In desperation, Gawain tells the lady that she must make the choice herself. This, of course, is the required outcome; as soon as he presents her with her own choice, the spell is broken and his wife remains a beautiful woman by night and by day.

The answer to both Arthur's riddle and Gawain's question is the same; a woman must be true to her own nature or, in the words of Arthur's reply to the knight, must 'get her own way'! What a woman most wants is to be accepted as herself. Male society tends to cast women in a linear and stereotyped image, ignoring their cyclic nature. By being given her own choice between the two poles of her nature, the Loathly Lady was able to absorb all aspects of it and become a beautiful, balanced woman. It is important to note that in both cases it is the men who must be made aware of this fact. In western society, a woman is rarely allowed to be true to her nature and it is necessary for her to pose the riddle to men in order to awaken their understanding.

In *Snow White*, the darker feminine aspect appears in the story as the wicked stepmother, with Snow White herself as the bright virgin. In the original story the wicked stepmother / queen appears as a mature, beautiful, experienced woman in full control of her magical powers of womanhood. In the guise of an old woman, she offers Snow White an apple which has been poisoned on the red side – the colour is significant. The queen takes on the role of initiator; she destroys the girl-child and offers the powers of menstruation through the red apple.

Having bitten into the apple, Snow White – believed to be dead – is placed in a glass coffin which is visited by three birds; an owl, a raven and a dove. The owl has long been associated with death, the wisdom of the subconscious and self-realization. The raven is also a bird of death and the dove symbolizes enlightenment.

Snow White is later 'awoken' by a prince, who makes her his wife and queen. She is no longer the virgin child but a woman who has awoken to her full sexual and creative energies, through her menstruation. Thus the entire story can be seen as an allegory for initiation into adult life, sexuality and, ultimately, the *Mother* phase.

It is interesting also to note that at the beginning of the story Snow White's mother sits sewing by an ebony framed window. As she gazes out at the falling snow flakes she pricks her finger with her sewing needle and the drops of blood fall onto the snow. The blood looks so beautiful that she makes a wish for a child who will be as white as snow, as red as blood and as black as ebony. Soon afterwards, she gives birth to a girl whose skin is as white as snow, whose lips are as red as blood and whose hair is as black as ebony. The colours are significant, as they are those of the triple goddess aspects of a woman's life.

In the story of Snow White, all three aspects of the triple goddess make an appearance, as well as the fourth aspect of enchantress. Snow White at first represents the Maiden, with her true mother representing the Mother. The wicked stepmother takes on two roles; firstly she plays the role of the beautiful Enchantress and then, in disguise as an old apple seller, she plays the Crone.

The story of *Sleeping Beauty* can also be seen to be menstrually orientated. Within *Sleeping Beauty*, the father, the king, tries to stop his daughter from growing up and becoming a woman. At the birth of his daughter, he invites the wise women from his kingdom to attend a celebration. Unfortunately he only has twelve gold plates and there are thirteen wise women and so the king neglects to invite the least attractive and most ugly of the women. At the feast, each wise woman in turn stands to give the child a gift which will enhance her life. As the twelfth woman stands the thirteenth, uninvited, storms into the hall and pronounces a prophecy that the child will prick her finger on a spindle in her fifteenth year and die. Although the final wise woman does not have the power to cancel the prophecy, she is able to soften it by making the child fall asleep for a hundred years, rather than dying.

The thirteen wise women represent the lunar year and by leaving out the thirteenth, the king is preventing the rhythm of nature from completing its natural cycle. As the uninvited woman prophesies, the inevitable penalty for this is death, the stopping of growth.

In a hopeless attempt to alter the prophecy, the king bans all spindles from his kingdom – in this way he feels that he can keep his daughter safe. The spindle is a symbol of the cycling rhythms of the universe and of the spiralling progression of the thread of life. By banning the spindles, the king is once more trying to halt the natural progress of life and prevent his daughter from starting menstruation and becoming a woman.

In her fifteenth year, as foreseen, the princess is lured into a neglected tower room where she meets an unfamiliar old woman sitting spinning. The girl pricks her finger on the spindle and immediately falls asleep. Once again the old woman or crone acts as initiator of menstruation and the term 'pricking a finger' is used to describe the princess's first menstrual blood. It is significant that this occurs in the girl's fifteenth year; not only was this a common age for the onset of menstruation, but the fifteenth day of the moon's cycle is the time of the full moon. The girl is no longer a maiden; she has reached maturity and begins the transition into the darkness of the waning moon, menstruation and womanhood.

The princess becomes suspended outside time and a thorn hedge grows around the castle, isolating it from the world. When a hundred years have passed, the instrument of the princess's awakening, as in *Snow White*, is a prince. The prince is allowed through the hedge and awakens the newly menstrual princess with a kiss.

This story looks not only at the change from child into womanhood, but also at the relationship between the father and the daughter's menstruation. The father's fear of the daughter growing up, becoming a woman and then looking to another male is shown by his attempts to stop her growth into womanhood.

In the story *The Awakening*, the Red Lady represents the faces of the evil stepmother, the thirteenth wise woman and the Loathly Lady. She is the initiator, who awakens the darker energies and understanding within Eve. Here the term 'dark' is used to represent empowering, accumulating, 'inner' energies rather than inherently destructive or evil ones. The Moon Lady represents the vitalizing and nurturing powers of womanhood and she guides Eve towards awareness of her cycle and its energies. The Moon Lady is the true mother of Snow White and the beautiful version of the Loathly Lady, and like the Loathly Lady, she absorbs both sides of the cycle to become a single, balanced woman at the end of the story. Eve, of course, plays the part of the Maiden and she represents all women who seek knowledge of their true nature.

THE HOLDER OF MEASURE

The development of the menstrual cycle was an important event in the evolution of womankind to a stage beyond the animal kingdom. Through the menstrual cycle, women became capable of arousal and thus sexually active throughout the month, rather than being limited to seasonal periods of being 'on heat'. During the month, women experienced highs in sexuality and creativity at both ovulation and menstruation, allowing them access to the creative energies which in animals were only available for purposes of procreation. In women, this creative energy at times when they were not physically fertile offered the procreation of ideas rather than new life.

The experience of the menstrual cycle and its parallels with the cycle of the moon brought the first concepts of measurement and time. Since the beginning of humankind, the body and its interaction with things around it has been used as the fundamental unit of measure. For example, the length of the foot on the ground or the amount of ground covered by a single pace became measures for distance. From the concepts of sequence and measurement came the division of time and the first clocks and calendars. Many cultures measured their time in nights and lunar months, setting their religious festivals by the full moon. Even today, the date of the Christian festival of Easter is determined by the occurrence of the full moon, as are many festivals in the Islamic and Jewish religions.

The concept of the link between women and their menstruation, the

moon, measurement and wisdom, is found reflected in many cultures
throughout the world and in many languages. The word *menstruation* is
derived from the Latin word for month, which itself also means moon.
These ideas found expression in the whole range of activities leading
to the building of civilization; in agriculture, social organization, arts
and crafts, commerce, learning, prophecy and religion. Many surviving
images and mythologies of early goddesses depict them as teaching
humanity these skills and abilities. On this basis, menstruation was
not a 'curse' given to women, but rather a gift from which sprang the
structure and variety of human culture. The image of the moon as
a reflection of the woman's cycle became a symbol of the creative
energies which she embodied.

The synchronicity of the woman's cycle and that of the moon also
reflected the link between the woman and the divine. Through the
woman's cycle, she carried the mystery of life within her body and
she was able to create life and ensure the future of her people. By
bringing the unmanifest into the world of creation, each woman held
the lifegiving, sustaining, creative powers of the universe.

Similar symbolism was found in the image of the spider. Just as the
spider weaves her web from within her body, the spider goddess was
seen as the creator of the web of space and time, bringing structure
and life to all of creation and being aware at the same time of each
vibration within the web. As the Lady of the Net, she spun the
threads of life and wove them into the patterns and fabric of all living
things. Later goddesses were associated with the skills of spinning and
weaving, not only as patronesses of the craft, but as representatives of
the spinning of life and death. The spinning goddess spun the thread
of an individual from the fibres of life, the Mother wove the tapestry
of experience, time cut the threads and the dark goddess unravelled
the tapestry back into its constituent fibres to spin again.

The menstrual cycle of a woman's womb was seen as a cycle of life
and fertility at ovulation and of death and infertility at menstruation;
a cycle which was represented in the moon's phases and was also a
reflection of the land's seasons. In many mythologies this mystery of
the womb is represented by the image of a magical or transforming
vessel. In the Grail legends it takes on the shape of a cup or grail;
in early Celtic mythology, it takes the form of a cauldron and in
later alchemical texts it takes the form of the flask or alembic. These
vessels each offered abundance, fertility, life, transformation, spiritual
inspiration and initiation.

The Grail legends in particular offered understanding and awareness
of the energies of the womb and of the menstrual cycle of women. The
Holy Grail was purported to be the cup of Christ used at the Last Supper

and later held by Joseph of Arimathea to catch the blood flowing from the dying Christ's wounds. It was a source of life and death as well as of spiritual inspiration, for those who attained it would die in this world, to be reborn into the next. The Grail could offer white wine or red; like the womb it offered the powers of ovulation and menstruation, of life and death.

The women in the Grail stories did not hunt for the Grail because the Grail, that is, the powers of the divine feminine, already resided within their own nature. Throughout the stories, the female characters reflect the aspects and energies of the divine feminine, not as many different women but as many different aspects of the same woman. The Grail legends reveal to women their own true nature, and, as bearers of the Grail, the need for them to acknowledge all aspects of its energies within themselves and to express these in the world.

In the story *The Awakening*, the Holder of Measure is an image of all menstruating women. She came into being with the shedding of the first menstrual blood and she holds the rhythm of women until the last. She symbolizes the power of time, of creative energies, of civilization and of life itself. Once a month she sheds a salt tear, 'the water of life', an egg and a drop of blood, 'the source of life', into a grail, the womb.

THE WOMB TREE

There are two major images used in mythology and legend to symbolize the feminine energies; the first is the cup or grail, symbolizing the regenerative, transformative potential and the second is the tree or pillar, symbolizing the dynamic, inspirational, ecstatic energies. The image of the sacred moon tree is very ancient and appears repeatedly in religious art from sources as diverse as early Assyrian cultures to the medieval and modern Christian Church.

In Assyrian art, the moon tree was depicted as laden with fruits, with a crescent moon riding above the branches, although this image was sometimes stylized to a pillar topped by the moon. As well as fruits, the moon tree was often depicted adorned with lights or ribbons, an image which is familiar in modern times in the Christmas tree or the maypole. The maypole may be regarded as a stylized moon tree, with the circle dance of the white, red and blue ribbons weaving the different feminine energies to bring about the spring fertility.

Many lunar goddesses were linked with a particular tree, some of which were magical and some of common or mundane species. In Greek mythology, the goddess Athene represented the creative fire of inspiration and was represented by the dark-fruited olive tree. The Greek Tree of Life bore golden apples and was called Hera's tree after the goddess of the moon at dawn and at dusk, whose name meant 'womb'.

The apple tree also appears in numerous legends and stories as a tree which bears the fruit of life and as a source of menstrual wisdom. The stories of Snow White and Adam and Eve both show the apple tree's fruit bearing the awakening of menstruation and the 'curse' of death. In the medieval *Vita Merlini*, the Life of Merlin, an apple woman appears as the bringer of death through her fruit. Rejected by the young Merlin, the apple woman tries to exact revenge later in his life by offering him her poisonous apples to eat. Although Merlin escapes this fate, his companions eat the apples and are driven mad. In Arthurian legend, King Arthur, mortally wounded at the battle of Camlann, was carried by Morgan La Fey to Avalon, the otherworld Island of Apples, to be healed.

Another tree having red fruit and strong moon tree imagery is the rowan. The rowan is also called the quickbeam, the mountain ash or the witchwood. The name quickbeam means 'tree of life'. Alongside the hazel and the apple, the rowan fruit was considered to be the food of the gods and it was taboo to eat the bright red berries. The colour red has very ancient associations with the energies of life; it represented the life blood, the blood of birth, the blood of fertility and the blood of menstruation. Like the Womb Tree, the rowan's branches are laden with clusters of bright red fruit and its powers were believed to be those of the creative energies, of inspiration, prophecy, healing and divination.

In *The Awakening*, the Womb Tree is a personal image of the sacred moon tree, the tree of life and knowledge. Shaped like the womb, holding the fruits of life and the form of the moon in its branches, it provides a conscious link between a woman, the energies of her cycle and the moon. The waters of the Womb Tree are the waters of a woman's subconscious; they are the inner source of creative inspiration and from these waters ideas and intuition are given birth. Water has always had strong links with the inner world and early worshippers offered prayers of thanks or supplication by throwing a votive offering into water. By visualizing the Womb Tree and throwing a request into the water, a woman can form a link with her creative source and give birth to idea children. The use of the Womb Tree in visualization will be approached in more detail in Chapter 4.

The fruit of the Womb Tree holds the knowledge and the life-bestowing power of the menstrual cycle and the rhythms of life. By picking the fruit, Eve awakens those rhythms within herself, activating the relationship between her mind, her womb and her creative energies. The fruit, however, cannot be taken without also taking the serpent, as it is the experience of the serpent and its renewing energies which brings the knowledge of the menstrual cycle.

THE SERPENT

The serpent appears in mythology as perhaps the most powerful of all images of renewal and transformation. It is the guardian of the wisdom of the underworld and of prophecy. The ability of the snake to regularly shed its old skin and renew itself was reflected each month in the renewal of the new moon and in the menstrual cycle of women. Like the moon, the snake was seen as a symbol of light and of darkness; it lived both above the ground and in the earth in burrows and caves. It represented the powers of the dark moon, the dynamic energy which arose from the inner consciousness or underworld and which brought into the light the powers of prophecy, wisdom, inspiration and fertility. The snake's sinuous, ripplelike movements reinforced its association with water and it became a symbol of the waters of heaven as fertilizing rain, the waters of the earth as lifegiving rivers and the waters of the underworld as the womb which brought rebirth and new life.

In some mythologies the snake represented the creative source which gave birth to the universe. The serpent was seen as the dynamic energy of the goddess who was both the earth-womb and that power within the earth which made the plants grow.

Many goddesses were linked to snakes. In some cases, this may indicate that these deities were originally seen in terms of the whole of the moon's cycle, rather than the single phase with which they later became associated.

Hel, the Teutonic goddess of the underworld and the dead, was the sister of the world serpent Uroboros, which encircled the oceans of the earth. Both Inanna and Ishtar were depicted with serpents, often intertwined around a staff, and were called the Queen of the Upper and Lower Waters. In the sanctuary at Knossos on Crete, statues were found of goddesses or priestesses with snakes wrapped around their bodies and in their hands. Hecate, the Greek dark moon goddess, was depicted with snakes in her hair, and Demeter, goddess of the corn, was attended by a snake.

In particular, goddesses who were patrons of learning, oracle, healing, wisdom and inspiration were associated with snakes. The priestess of Artemis was called the 'pythia' or serpent and her shrine was a place of healing and prophecy. Athene's shield and the *aegis*, a garment which she wore across her shoulders, were both adorned with pictures of the snakehaired Gorgon's head and the aegis was also fringed with snakes. In Celtic legend, the goddess Brigid was particularly associated with snakes and the snakeheaded Egyptian goddess, Heh, was called the Revealer of Wisdom.

Serpents are also found in mythology and legend guarding the tree of life. The tree as an image of the goddess brought union between the earth, heaven and underworld, through which the energies of life poured in the symbol of the snake. The serpent was the rising and falling sap, the living, dying, renewing aspect of the eternal source of life. The imagery of the story of Adam and Eve is similar to that found in Mesopotamia, Egypt and other cultures in which the divine feminine was represented. The tree of life, whose rhythmic shedding and rebirth of its leaves each year echoed the rhythms of the snake, the moon and women, was an image of death followed by rebirth. The story of Adam and Eve has two trees, the tree of life and the tree of knowledge, separating the concept of an individual's awareness of the cycle of life and rebirth from the cycle of nature. Eve, however, rejoins these ideas with the picking of the fruit. By taking the fruit, she takes on the cyclic nature of menstruation; she becomes linked to the rhythms of nature and of the universe, aware on a personal level of the interconnectedness of these rhythms and the cycle of life.

This gift, which should be seen as bringing knowledge of life, death and rebirth through a woman's cycle, was instead ultimately perceived as a symbol of betrayal, of womankind bringing death and evil into the world. Eve's menstruation and subsequent expulsion from Eden became the root cause of mortal death, a death which was seen as an end rather than part of a continuing cycle. The gift became twisted further, so that the sexuality and fertility which came with the woman's cycle were also regarded as sinful and that by being born of the womb all human life inherited the evil existing in the womb, the 'original sin'. The gift of womanhood became 'the curse' of womanhood.

Although there is no mention of the story in the Bible, many traditions hold that Eve was in fact Adam's second wife. His first wife, Lilith, was created as Adam's equal and fled from Eden when her sexuality was denied. Unlike Eve, Lilith already possessed all the powers of womanhood. Lilith came to epitomize the destroyer, the temptress and death, all the aspects of the dark moon feared by patriarchal society and denied to the initial 'good' and innocent image of Eve. In later legend, Lilith became an aggressive sexual temptress, the consort of Satan, with domain over basic instincts and carnal pleasure. In medieval art, she was the serpent coiled around the tree of life, often depicted with the same face as Eve. By 'tempting' her, Lilith awoke within Eve her own menstrual cycle, unlocking the knowledge which it holds of light and darkness, and making her, in the eyes of men, 'bad' like Lilith.

After biting the apple herself, Eve offered the fruit to Adam and in doing so she offered the awareness and knowledge of the tree of life through herself. In other stories and legends, men are told that they must not pick the fruit from the tree of life because it is poisonous to them. In a medieval Scottish faery tale, this warning was given to the mortal Thomas the Rhymer by the faery queen who abducted him and carried him off into the otherworld. The fruit of menstruation cannot be picked by men, as it holds the knowledge intrinsic to the rhythmic nature of women; but its gifts may be given to men by women who have themselves picked the fruit. This powerful and important symbolism in the Adam and Eve story was replaced with the derogatory image of women being weaker in nature than men and the source of man's temptation away from the divine rather than towards it.

In some cultures it was believed that a girl's first act of sex was with a snake and that this caused menstruation. In others, it was a snake's bite which started the bleeding. Both Eve in *The Awakening* and Eve in the garden of Eden awoke to their womanhood through the intervention of the serpent. The knowledge of life presented by the fruit and inherent in womanhood cannot be received without also accepting the rhythmic sexual and creative energies of the serpent.

MOON ANIMALS

Animals play an important part in legends and mythology, where they are often portrayed as having magical abilities. These stories hide a wealth of information, the understanding of which has been virtually lost to modern society. Animal images have become 'cute', sanitized or labelled simply as children's story characters.

Many of the animals found in old stories and legend, however, have strong lunar associations and are often found linked to women or goddesses. They play an important part in the stories, either by offering teaching or guidance or by representing the energies of the woman or goddess in a form to which a person can relate on a non-intellectual level. Some animals represent a particular facet of a goddess; in some cases, an aspect which has lost importance or been hidden. Others embody the underlying energies of women or of the moon.

These animals are not just part of a story, they are images which obtain reality in our minds and imaginations. They represent the instinctual level of our being, a level which is important to women but which is repressed by the modern, scientifically orientated world.

It is not practical in a book such as this to examine all animals which have lunar or female associations but it is worth looking at a few of the more obvious ones, and a few not so obvious.

The Butterfly

The use of the butterfly as a symbol of femininity goes back even as far as neolithic times. The image of the butterfly represented the Minoan goddess of life and fertility, echoing in the shape of its wings the labia outlining the entrance to a woman's vagina. In Aztec culture, the butterfly was used as a symbol of fertility and vegetation and a particular species of butterfly was a symbol of the goddess in rites associated with women and flowers.

The butterfly was associated with the soul and the fire of spirit and rebirth. The transformation from caterpillar to butterfly was seen as a metaphor for the concept of life after death, leaving the old earthbound body for a new and more beautiful form. In Irish legend the maiden Etain was changed by a rival in love into the form of a butterfly and travelled around the world in this shape until she was reborn once more in human form. The butterfly was also associated with fire and the Gaelic word for the brand which lit the community's fires from the ceremonial bonfire is the same as that for 'butterfly'.

As with other female images, the butterfly was linked to the moon, the curve of its wings reflecting the crescents of the waxing and waning moon; the shape was stylized in the Minoan culture into the image of the doubleheaded axe or *labrys*.

The Unicorn

The unicorn was regarded as a creature of the moon. It was wise and beautiful, representing purity, gentleness and guardianship, and was the initiator of womanhood. There are many descriptions of the unicorn, with reports of the body shape and size varying from that of a goat to a large stag, but most enduring is the image of a pure white horse bearing a single horn on its forehead. The horn, which could be either spiralled or straight, was called the 'alicorn' and has been described as being white at the base, black in the middle and red at the tip, colours associated with female lunar figures. The alicorn had the ability to protect and to render any poison harmless, reflecting its power to transform. In Roman mythology, the unicorn was associated with the huntress Diana, who rode a chariot drawn by eight unicorns.

The unicorn was seen as a noble and intelligent beast, which lived alone in the wild woods as guardian and protector of the other woodland creatures. Too savage and dangerous to hunt in the normal manner, the only way to capture a unicorn was to lure it into a trap, using as bait a maiden, sometimes sitting willingly and ornately dressed, at other times unwillingly tied to a tree and naked. Attracted by the purity of the maiden, the unicorn would lay its head in the young girl's lap and allow itself to be captured or killed. The red tip of the unicorn's horn of transformation lying in the maiden's lap can be seen as a symbol of menstruation and the awakening of puberty and sexual experience.

The unicorn brought the first blood to the maiden, offering the spiralling cycle through the phases and colours of the moon. The unicorn was not lured by the maiden, but rather it brought to all maidens the gift of womanhood. The phallic symbol of the horn may hint that, like the serpent, the unicorn was considered to be a woman's first sexual partner, who brought on her bleeding.

Men could never catch the unicorn in the hunt because it repre-sented the lunar powers of womanhood, but once captured by the maiden, the unicorn could safely be led by her, as it was then a part of herself. The hunt for the unicorn may echo the hunt for the Holy Grail, which could only be found by men with the help of women. One belief held that every time a unicorn died, a little magic left the world. In the modern world, where the female energies of womanhood have been repressed, there are few unicorns. Perhaps it is time to call them back.

The Dove

Many moon goddesses are also depicted as bird goddesses and the dove in particular has long been associated with the divine feminine and with the moon. It was a symbol of Ishtar, Astarte, Inanna, Rhea, Demeter, Persephone, Venus, Aphrodite and Isis and became a representation of the Holy Grail. The dove is also found in many pictures of the Virgin Mary. Universally, the dove was a symbol of the queen of heaven, of femininity, gentleness, love, sexuality, spirituality, wisdom and peace.

As a symbol of the light of the moon, the dove brought wisdom and inspiration into the world. In gnostic tradition, Sophia, the 'Holy

Wisdom' of God, was represented by the dove, which was seen as bringing the light of the heavenly mother to earth. In medieval Christian art the dove represented the Holy Spirit and was pictured hovering over the head of Mary at the Annunciation and over Christ at his baptism.

The dove was also associated with the moon tree and doves were often portrayed sitting in the branches of the tree. A similar image can be found in depictions of the dove sitting in the hair of a moon goddess. The dove with an olive twig in its mouth offering the fruit of the tree was an emblem of the renewal of life for both Ishtar and Athene.

As well as being sacred to goddesses, white turtle doves were also sacred to the Fates, reflecting the link between the birds and lunar powers of prophecy and oracle. The ancient oracle at Dodona was an oak tree in which lived a flock of doves attended by a number of priestesses who were themselves called 'doves'. The oracle was found in the voices of the birds, in the sound of their rustling amongst the leaves or in their flight. In the paintings of the Annunciation, the dove is sometimes shown with its head towards Mary's ear, as though telling her of her fate.

The dove symbolized the aspect of the moon which bestowed life and love. It represented the ability of the female nature to bring harmony in the reuniting of the spirit with consciousness, humanity and nature and the inner voice of wisdom and intuition.

The Horse

In many cultures the horse, and in particular the mare, represented the powers of fertility, life energy, prophecy, magic and emotional and instinctual depths. A white mare especially symbolized the powers of the moon and her crescent-shaped horseshoes brought luck and protection. The mare symbolized motherhood, love and the fertility of the land. As the power of the land she held sovereignty and in Ireland the horse was used as part of their kingmaking rites. At harvest the corn spirit was thought to take the form of a horse.

Even in modern times the image of the horse, in the form of the hobby horse, can still be found displayed at the great turning points of the year. The hobby horse is usually a costume made for one person to wear and is often coloured black, red or white.

To the Celtic race the horse held great importance. The Gallic horse goddess Epona was a triple goddess often depicted seated on a mare, or with mares and foals, holding a cornucopia, a comb, a mirror or a goblet. The Welsh horse goddess Rhiannon owned a flock of birds whose singing could wake the dead or put the living to sleep, echoing the darker aspect of the goddess as goddess of death and rebirth.

The horse was linked to lakes and to the sea as well as to the land. The mare represented the Great Mother of the primordial waters, the source of all life. Even today the white foaming crests of waves are referred to as 'white horses'. Water was associated with the Celtic otherworld and in legend magical horses would carry heroes across the sea to this fabulous land. Folk stories tell of magical horses which grazed the banks of lakes and pools; if anyone attempted to ride these beasts, they would plunge the rider into the water, drowning or eating him. In some stories the horses could be identified by the fact that their hooves and horseshoes were back-to-front. These water horse images reflect the dark moon aspects of death and transportation into the inner depths.

Horses held the link between the visible and invisible worlds and were ridden by shamans who could travel between the two. The horse was also one of the animals into which it was commonly held that a witch could transform herself.

In one image, the horse symbolizes the complete lunar cycle. It represents the dynamic forces of life and the manifest fertility of the visible moon phases, and at the same time it represents the hidden, inner powers of transformation and death of the dark moon.

The Crane

The crane is not a bird which is immediately associated with many folk stories or legends. In Greek mythology it was seen as a guardian and a symbol of vigilance and patience and in Celtic lore it had strong female associations. The European crane is a large grey bird with a long white neck, a black head and a bright red cap. As a water bird it was linked to the otherworld and was seen as a secret and magical beast with dark powers.

In Celtic legend the crane was associated with hostile goddesses, old women and ill-tempered or sexually promiscuous women. There are a number of stories in which women are transformed into cranes: St Columba of Ireland turned a queen and her handmaidens into cranes as a punishment, the sea god Mannanan possessed a magical bag made from the skin of a crane which had formerly been a woman, transformed because of her jealousy, and the Irish hero Fionn was rescued from falling over a cliff as a child by his grandmother, who had transformed herself into a crane.

The crane was also associated with death and with the death of the old year and the turning of the seasons. Irish stories tell of the 'four cranes of death', who were the enchanted sons of an old woman called 'the hag of the temple'. The god Midir had three cranes who could rob warriors of their courage and fighting ability and if a warrior saw a crane on his way to battle, it was a very bad omen. This weakening of the warrior spirit attributed to the crane demonstrates taboos very similar to those associated with menstruating women.

In all these stories, crane women show behaviour and abilities akin to those of premenstrual and menstrual women. They are seen as rude, hostile, sexual and able to bring death and disaster to men. The crane, however, was also linked to prophecy, the turning of cycles, the inner reflective trance and guardianship, thus representing the positive aspects of these phases.

The Owl

In modern times, the owl has become a symbol of wisdom through its association with the Greek goddess Athene and the Roman goddess Minerva, but its older symbolism, which is carried through in country lore, associated it with death and destruction. The call of the owl in daylight, or heard three nights in a row, was believed to herald a death. In Scotland the owl was known as the *cailleach* or old woman, who was associated with death and winter.

The owl also has strong sexual imagery. In Wales it is said that the sound of an owl calling signified that an unmarried maiden had just lost her virginity. In Celtic legend, the owl appears in the story of Lleu. Lleu's magician uncles made for him a magical bride from flowers and plants and named her Blodeuwedd, that is 'Face of Flowers' in Welsh. Blodeuwedd, however, was faithful to Lleu for only as long as the flowers kept their fragrance and fell in love with a hunter. This hunter grievously wounded Lleu with a spear and he was close to death when found and cured by his uncles. In punishment for her betrayal, the unfaithful bride was turned into an owl and even today the name for an owl in the Welsh language is *Blodeuwedd*.

Blodeuwedd was a sexual woman who followed her own nature; in many ways, the blame for the betrayal was not hers but that of the men who created her with unrealistic expectations. The story of Blodeuwedd is similar to that of Lilith who was made, as Adam was, from the earth. As she was his equal, she refused to couple with him lying on her back and fled from Eden. Lilith became associated with the screech owl and was depicted with clawed feet and bird wings. She was seen as demonic, the dark aspect of the moon and of womanhood. She was the queen of the underworld, bringer of death to babies and the seducer of men in the night. As such she was the dark aspect of Eve, the menstrual curse which Eve brought into the world through the serpent.

Both stories show the true nature of women, to progress from the maiden to the crone. The owl symbolized the dark inner powers and wisdom of the menstrual cycle and the necessary transformation and death of the old self to bring about renewal.

The Hare

Hares, and later rabbits, were symbols of fertility, the dynamic energy of life, growth, renewal and sexual pleasure, and were closely associated with the moon and its goddesses. In particular, the hare was associated with the goddess Oestra, who gave her name to the modern festival of Easter. Oestra was depicted as having a hare's head and it was her hares who laid the eggs of new life to herald the birth of spring – an image which can still be found in the modern 'easter bunny'.

The Norse moon goddess and Freyja, goddess of love and fecundity, were both attended by hares, as was the Roman goddess Venus. The patterns on the face of the full moon are said to portray a rabbit or hare and in eastern tradition the hare gets its fertility from gazing up at the moon.

The hare was also associated with the lunar/female powers of divination, transformation, inspired madness and sexuality. The Celtic queen Boudicca kept a hare for divination, releasing it from beneath her cloak before battle and using its path as it ran to predict the outcome.

The association of the hare with sexuality has survived into modern times and has found expression in the concept of the 'bunny girl'. It is possible that because of these 'undesirable' aspects, the medieval Church viewed the hare as a beast of ill omen. Hares became associated with witches and a witch in hare's form could only be killed with a silver crucifix or, later, a silver bullet.

THE DARK GODDESS

The prehistoric image of the source of life was that of a goddess who was seen as *both* the transforming womb and as the dynamic, generative forces which created the universe and all life. She was viewed as the continuous, invisible life force of the universe and creation was her manifest body.

The expression of this imagery was observed in the cycle of the moon and its phases. The goddess was seen as manifest in the three light phases of the moon as a trinity of growth, fruition and decay, reflecting the transient cycle of the seasons and of life. The unmanifest goddess was the dark phase of the moon, the womb, the invisible, continuous source of life. Later depictions of the moon goddess showed her as a trinity rather than in four-fold aspect not because the dark aspect was unknown, but because she was hidden to the human eye like the dark phase of the moon. She was the darkness of the invisible, unmanifest, the source of life and potential, and was the pure consciousness which lay behind the trinity of light. Her darkness was the essence of the whole cycle, as the light phases could not be perceived except in relationship to the darkness.

The image of the goddess of life and death, darkness and light as the whole cycle of the moon became split, with the image of the dark goddess of destructive energies and death becoming separated from her other aspect of generative energies and life. The female image of death and destruction was no longer followed by the compensating image of the return to the universal womb to be reborn and thus the lunar cycle of life, death and rebirth was broken. The image of the divine feminine became polarized into the bright goddess of life and the terrifying, underworld goddess who brought the finality of death.

The powerful sexuality and destructive energies experienced by women in their menstrual cycles were brought together in the image of bloodlusting war goddesses. The creative aspect of the energies was ignored and the wild, bloodcrazed sexual image was expressed in goddesses like Ishtar, Sekhmet and the Morrigan. The welcoming mother of death became perceived as evil, dealing in senseless and wanton destruction. This linking of 'sex and violence' has continued into modern society, reflected in films and books and in the number of violent rapes of women. The original image, of creative sexuality and death intertwined, has become horribly distorted. The Destroyer as the bringer of change is frightening if viewed from a linear perspective, but if life and death are viewed as a continual cycle, the Destroyer becomes the way to a new existence and new growth.

Mythology has often restricted goddesses to the good 'mother of life' or to the frightening 'goddess of death' aspects but often the images still hold remnants of the whole cycle. Hecate, the Greek goddess of the dark moon, was the queen of witches and a goddess of death. As the waning and dark aspect of the moon, she was the patron of divination, dreams and magic and was the force which arose out of the inner darkness to bring visions, compulsions, ecstatic inspiration and destructive madness. As the queen of the dead, Hecate held the torch of regeneration and rebirth. In other stories, Hecate was described as wearing a bright headband and being tenderhearted; it was Hecate who offered compassion to the grieving Demeter after the abduction of Persephone. She was worshipped as a triple image and at crossroads, where the four paths reflected the four phases of the moon. Approaching a crossroads, you may see the three paths in front, but the fourth path is hidden beneath your feet.

The goddess Athene, who was a virgin goddess of wisdom and intellect, also carried images of her darker aspect. The Gorgon's head was closely associated with Athene, being pictured on her shield or on her aegis. In legend, the Gorgon was Medusa, a woman with snakes for her hair whose deadly gaze turned men to stone. Her blood had the power to kill or to renew, depending on which vein it came from. The fact that her face was surrounded by writhing snakes, reflecting the image of the vulva, made her a symbol of sexuality, regeneration, creation, renewal and death. Athene was also depicted with the owl, with its associations with death and the powers of prophecy.

Both Hecate and Athene can thus be seen to contain the image of other aspects of the moon's phases to some degree in a single goddess image.

The descent of a goddess into the realm of the dead to bring back new life and knowledge is a recurrent theme in mythology and reflects the cycle of the seasons, the moon and of women. In Greek legend, Persephone, the daughter of the corn goddess Demeter, was abducted into the underworld. Demeter in her grief withdrew the powers of fertility and growth from the world until her daughter should be found. Persephone could only return completely to the world above if she took nothing from the underworld, but she ate some pomegranate seeds, an act which bound her to return to the underworld once a year.

Persephone, or Kore, was the Maiden of the corn plant, the seed, whilst Demeter was the corn itself. The story echoes the uniting principle of the moon's cycle, where the child of the mother is of the same substance as the mother. The cutting of the corn and its death did not kill that which made the corn grow, but was necessary for it to be brought back to life. Persephone, as the corn seed, rested in the underworld until she was reborn in the spring and for that part of the year she was the queen of the dead.

The descent of Persephone can also be seen as reflecting the cycle of women, as well as the cycle of life. Once a month, women withdraw into the waning phase of their monthly cycles to rest in the darkness of menstruation. Persephone, like Eve, takes the red fruit of menstruation and becomes linked to a cycle of withdrawal, renewal of energies and descent into the underworld. Above her in the world the energies of fertility are withdrawn into winter by Demeter, reflecting the sympathy between a woman's cycle and that of the land. At menstruation a woman experiences a withdrawal of her energies from the outside world, focusing her awareness inwards to aid her own growth and understanding so that she can bring the knowledge out into the everyday world. Both Persephone and the menstruating woman are in a state of winter, with the fertile energies withdrawn. The first descent into darkness is necessary for a maiden to grow into a mother. The successive descents each month enable a woman to receive back into herself the younger part of herself, so that she can begin life again. To descend each month with Persephone is to descend into the underworld of the subconsciousness, to become closer to the source of all life and consciousness and to give meaning and understanding to life.

The story of *The Awakening* follows the path of Eve's first descent. The Red Lady is the Enchantress or wicked stepmother; she destroys the child in Eve by awakening her powers of womanhood. The Red Lady holds the powers of visions, of magic, transformation and truth. In the darkness, her vision brings Eve madness, compulsion, ecstatic inspiration, sexual and dynamic energies. Before these energies bring destruction through Eve and in Eve, she is called by the Mother of Darkness to transform her energies, creating out of destruction and bringing light out of darkness. By descending, Eve experiences the existence of two worlds, the everyday, visible world and the inner, invisible world. Like the prehistoric goddess, she is of both worlds and moves between the two each month. Her first descent starts the spiralling cycles of renewal which will accompany her through her fertile life.

SOVEREIGNTY

The stories of Celtic and later Arthurian legend often involved mystical women who appeared as the earthly representatives of the goddess of sovereignty or the land. As Sovereignty, these women were able to offer the gifts of creativity, wisdom and divine kingship. Through their marriage to the representative of the sovereignty of the land, the Celtic kings were given divine right to rule and their authority and the honour of their kingship were linked mythically with the goddess of the land.

The king was expected to guide his people and to be true to them, in return for which Sovereignty would offer him the powers and wisdom of the otherworld. In Irish kingmaking ceremonies, the Sovereignty of the land was represented by a white mare and in Arthurian legend she was represented by the triple form of Guinevere. The Welsh name Gwenhwyfar means 'White Phantom' and reflects the lunar quality of Sovereignty.

Sovereignty appears throughout these legends in the form of a number of women who each hold a lunar quality and manifest an aspect of the land and the divine feminine. Sovereignty takes on the guise of the inviting maiden, the bountiful queen, the hideous damsel or dark maiden and the old hag. These women appear to heroes and to kings, offering them gifts and teachings and setting them challenges which allow them to champion the cause of the land.

The maiden, whose colour is white, is portrayed as the source of vision, an initiator of action. A similar role can be found in other folk stories where maidens need to be rescued from dragons, monsters or evil witches and even today it is a theme found in books and films. Guinevere first took the role of the beautiful flower bride who was the source of sovereignty for Arthur, but when neglected by the king she became the vision of sovereignty for Lancelot.

Guinevere's role as queen in the earlier stories showed her as a woman who ruled the court and who sustained Arthur's position of power. The powerful and influential queen, whose colour was red, was often portrayed as enabling the hero to achieve his challenge or sustaining him on his quest. When her role as temporal queen was finished, Igraine, the mother of Arthur, retired to the otherworld where she maintained her role of power as the queen of the Castle of Maidens.

The dark maiden enters into the legends to actively challenge the hero, forcing him towards self-knowledge and responsible behaviour. In the Arthurian myths, she appeared as Kundry the sorceress, who reproached Peredur for not asking the Grail Question and goaded questing knights into action after scolding them for their inaction. She is portrayed as vicious with her tongue, testing and tormenting the knights.

The enchantress Morgan also reflected the dark maiden aspect in her antagonism towards King Arthur and in her constant challenging of his worthiness to be a king. The dark maiden could also be portrayed as the warrior-woman, whose role of companion was to teach and transform the hero's way of thinking. She held the power of magic and darkness, but she also represented the dynamism of the maiden.

The hag also appeared as a figure of darkness but she was seen as the holder of dark knowledge and transformation. She was often portrayed as being transformed from an old, ugly aspect into a young, beautiful maiden by the correct action of the hero, as seen in the story of Sir Gawain and the Loathly Lady.

These aspects of Sovereignty reflected the cycle of the moon; like the moon, the aspects of the maiden, mother, dark maiden and hag were not fixed, but were seen as changing and transforming from one to another. Sovereignty, as goddess of the land, reflected the nature of the land, the burgeoning energy of spring, the bounty of summer, the withdrawal of autumn and the darkness of winter where the manifest beauty of the land was hidden, but she also represented this cycle in her earthly representatives, in a woman's menstrual cycle.

As with the moon and seasons, a woman also flows from one aspect of her cycle to another, changing and transforming in tune with her nature. Sovereignty as the land inspires humankind, offers it her bounty, reproaches it for its inaction or wrong action and transforms the way we are.

Sovereignty may also appear in stories and myths as the 'ideal woman', whose appearance reflects all three of the lunar colours; white of skin, black of hair and red of lips, balancing all the colours and their symbolism within herself. She has self-knowledge and is true to her nature. In one version of the story of Gawain, the answer to the Black Knight's question was that a woman most desires to have 'sovereignty'. In context, this has a rather deeper meaning than 'getting her own way'!

The Arthurian legends show not only the different aspects of Sovereignty, but also the interactions between women and Sovereignty and between men and Sovereignty. For women, the quest for the Holy Grail, the cup of Sovereignty, lies within their own experience and their identification with each of the aspects of Sovereignty within themselves and their cycles. For men, however, only he who is just, honest, truthful and loving may hold the kingship of the land as the representative or partner of Sovereignty and in return she inspires, empowers, guides and teaches. An ordinary woman may also offer the same gifts to a man, but only if he recognizes the sovereignty within her and enables her to be true to her own sovereign nature. Sovereignty demands the freedom to be herself and this freedom has to be given by other women as well as men. The love and trust which a man gives a woman in allowing her sovereignty is returned in the gifts of her sovereignty.

THE FEMALE SHAMAN AND PRIESTESS

A woman who becomes aware of her cycle and of its energies learns also an awareness of a level of life beyond the visible. She holds an intuitive link with the energies of life, birth and death and perceives divinity within the land and within herself. From this awareness, the woman interacts not only with the visible and mundane but also with the invisible and spiritual aspects of her life.

It was through this monthly altered state of awareness that the female shamans/medicine woman, or later the priestess, brought her energies, insights and connection with the divine into the manifest world and to her community. Healing, magic, prophecy, teaching, inspiration and survival all came from her ability to feel both worlds, to travel between them and to bring her experiences from one to the other.

The increase in the dominance of men in society and religion led to the decline in the status of the female shaman and priestess, until ultimately men took over their positions and roles. The role of the priestess was repressed so thoroughly and completely that the active position of a woman in structured religion all but disappeared. The less structured position of the wise woman or witch was able to continue 'underground' and became the last link with the ancient matriarchal religions. The village witch was versed in the magic of nature, healing and relationships and was able to interact with her menstrual cycle, the seasons and her intuitive, inner self. She offered help and guidance in the passage of life and death, she brought initiation and transformation through the rites of passage and she led the ecstatic rites which brought connectedness, fertility and inspiration to her people.

The village witch offered the balance of female awareness and energies within male-dominated society and religion. Unfortunately, these powers of the feminine were also clearly seen as a threat to the male structure and the medieval witch persecutions virtually destroyed the traditions of the witch or wise woman in society. By attacking the witches, the persecutors acknowledged that these women had power, but the virtual destruction of the status of witchcraft resulted rather from society's later denial of these feminine powers. The witch became a object of ridicule, portrayed in children's books and at Hallowe'en as a comical figure. The early penalties for being caught and the later indoctrination of fear and shame deterred women from expressing the abilities and needs which would have reawakened the tradition. The direct effects of the witch persecutions are felt even today in the lack of any recognized spiritual teachings, archetypes or traditions in society which acknowledge the female nature and energies, let alone offer guidance in their use.

The result of the denial of active experience of their spirituality for women is that they themselves accept a male-structured and dominated religion, without any idea of their own innate spirituality. To become aware of this spirituality, a woman must stand outside the male religion and the majority of the religious community – an action which is very difficult if she has been brought up in a male religion without any concept of 'outside' and which can be very frightening due to the lack of tradition and guidance. The crushing of female-orientated spirituality is a comparatively recent event in the history of humankind but it was achieved so thoroughly that traces are left only in Western folklore, archaeology, myths and legends and in the need still felt within women.

With the rise of women's status in the twentieth century, there has been a growing need to express female spirituality in a recognized form. Under female pressure, some Christian Churches have accepted women into the priesthood, but although this acknowledges women as being spiritually aware, it negates their femininity. The term 'female priest', rather than 'priestess', makes the woman an 'honorary' male, ignoring the feminine nature and powers which she embodies. A woman cannot be a priest by virtue of her femininity, but it is *that very femininity* and sexuality which link her to the awareness of the divine, the rhythms of life and the universe. The priesthood offers women a *recognized* spiritual role, but it does not confer anything more. The ability to be a spiritual being is inherent in the nature and body of a woman.

The ability of the priestess/wise woman/female shaman/witch to mediate the powers of the divine is inherent in all women, and comes from a woman's awareness of herself. To become a priestess is to search within. The image of a woman holding a chalice has a different meaning from that of a man, whether this is recognized consciously or subconsciously, and perhaps it is this fact which frightens men into thinking that women will 'take over' their religion. There is a need to reawaken both images, which should be balanced and compatible, each accepted in its own right. The myth of the male and the myth of the female are not the same, but neither are they separate; they are intricately woven together in balance and harmony.

In the past, the moonlike nature of women was recognized as demonstrating the link between women and the universe. Through her body, the woman experienced intuitively the interconnectedness of all life, the lack of distinction between the divine and creation, and the cycle of life, death and rebirth. These realizations are missing from modern society and are difficult to comprehend unless they are experienced directly through the body for women and through women for men. There is no room in today's society for the ecstatic dances, spirituality expressed through sexuality and the body or the voice of prophecy or oracle. Society is cut off from the powers of the feminine, the inspiration and empathy which bring growth and understanding, the removal of the fear of death and the oneness of the mind, body, creation and the divine.

With the encroachment of the female into the 'male world' the advancement of women has been intellectual, empty of the intuitive understanding and creativity which is the basis of their nature. There are no archetypes or traditions to guide women on their needs and abilities in their new areas of work and experiences. It is therefore vitally important that women redress this lack and experience growth and recognition in society in all aspects of their nature.

The development of understanding in each individual woman is important and therefore the guidance of the passage from childhood into womanhood is also important. Modern society has lost many of its rites of passage and therefore there is a need to reinstate the rites of initiation at puberty, the seasonal and lunar rites and the rites of transformation at death and birth if society is to relearn the realizations of the menstrual cycle. New stories and myths need to be written, new songs sung and more archetypes painted if the tradition of women is to be re-established. The act of this reawakening reconnects women with their complete natures and offers that awareness to future generations in the hope that it will never be lost again. Most importantly, however, it creates a place in society for the female shaman, the wise woman, the oracular priestess, the witch, the medicine and spirit woman.

In *The Awakening*, Eve is acknowledged as being of two worlds and having the ability to walk between them. By carrying the red veil of menstruation, she holds in herself the powers and nature of the divine feminine. This responsibility accompanies her awakening into the realization of her true nature. For the modern woman who does not understand her cycle, the excuse of the menstrual cycle for behavioural problems is valid and even those who do understand their cycles are unable to accept responsibility because society does not let them express their true nature.

FOUR

Meeting the Moon

THE MENSTRUAL CYCLE

For most girls, their first menstruation starts at around the age of twelve and establishes a cycle of approximately twenty-eight days, although the length of the cycle may vary from fourteen to more than thirty days. The cycle will become a part of a woman's life until around the age of forty-seven, unless she becomes pregnant or suffers the loss of her period due to physiological factors.

Each month a woman's body undergoes a series of changes, many of which occur without her being consciously aware of them. These changes may include variations in hormone balances, vaginal temperature, urine composition and quantity, body weight, vitamin concentrations, water retention, heart rate, breast size and consistency, vaginal fluid consistency, concentration levels, vision and hearing, psychic ability, pain threshold and many others. It is important for each woman to become aware of how her body reacts to her own cycle if she is to understand the effect it has on her own personality and creative energies.

The monthly physical cycle consists of four phases: preovulatory, ovulatory, premenstrual and menstrual. Within each of a woman's ovaries are groups of cells called follicles which contain immature eggs or ova. During the *preovulatory* phase a follicle ripens, producing the hormone oestrogen which stimulates the breasts and the uterine wall (Figures 1 and 2). Around days 14–16 in the cycle the follicle bursts, releasing the egg; this is the *ovulation* phase. Some women are aware of certain physical symptoms which arise at ovulation; these may include a pain in the pelvic area, midcycle bleeding or spotting, increase in breast tenderness or size, or food cravings. After ovulation, the follicle becomes a 'corpus luteum' producing both progesterone and oestrogen. The progesterone prepares the uterine wall for fertilization.

Fallopian Tube
Ovary
Uterus
Cervix
Vagina

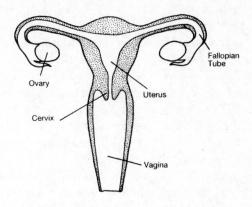

Figure 1. The Womb

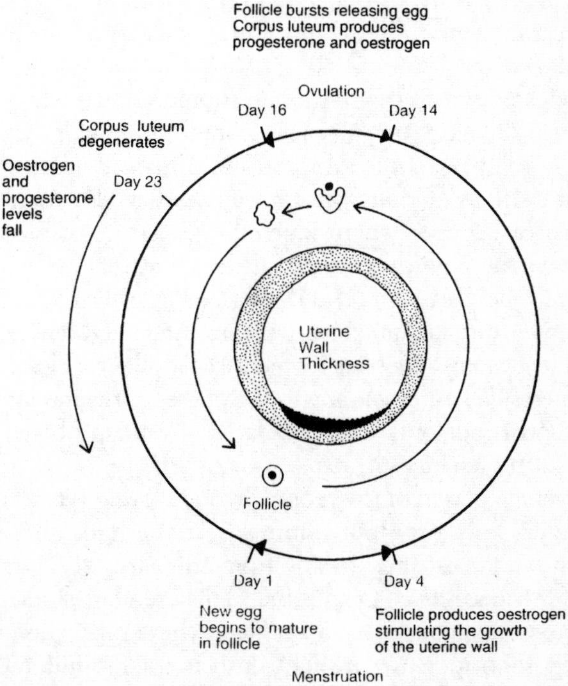

Follicle bursts releasing egg
Corpus luteum produces
progesterone and oestrogen
Ovulation
Day 16
Day 14
Corpus luteum
degenerates
Oestrogen
and
progesterone
levels
fall
Day 23
Uterine
Wall
Thickness
Follicle
Day 1
Day 4
New egg
begins to mature
in follicle
Follicle produces oestrogen
stimulating the growth
of the uterine wall
Menstruation

Figure 2. The Cycle of the Egg and Womb

If fertilization does not occur, the corpus luteum gradually degenerates and the levels of progesterone and oestrogen fall in the *premenstrual* phase. The uterine lining finally starts to disintegrate, starting the *menstrual* bleeding.

Physical and emotional premenstrual changes to women are now starting to be accepted by doctors, lawyers and judges and by employers. The variety of symptoms, though, is quite large and each can affect women to different degrees. Some of the most common symptoms are backache, fainting, migraine, sugar and carbohydrate cravings, breast tenderness and swelling, cystitis, cramps, water retention, fatigue, lack of concentration, allergies, irritability, mood swings, hostility and depression. A large percentage of all menstruating women experience premenstrual symptoms to some degree.

There are many physical means which may be used to help relieve these symptoms, ranging from vitamins and minerals in the diet to massage and aromatherapy, but none of these methods make use of the link which the woman already has with her own womb through her subconscious. The physical methods tend to treat the condition of menstruation as an illness of the body, separate from the mind. If a woman can learn to understand her cycle, to accept the changes and to become true to her own nature, she can regain the balance of her cycle.

This does not mean that a woman should not use whatever methods she can to alleviate any physical symptoms; it does mean that she should stop fighting these symptoms and instead accept them as part of herself. This is obviously not always easy to do when in the pit of a premenstrual low or when doubled over in the pain of bleeding!

Although the physical changes of the menstrual cycle are beginning to be more widely understood and discussed in society, the inner changes of sexuality, spirituality and creativity are still largely ignored. As already discussed, the moon and women's menstrual cycles are closely interlinked, with women's bodies responding to the phases of the moon; but the cycle of the moon is not only the calendar of a woman's body, it is also an indicator of the changes in her consciousness.

The average period of the moon's synodic cycle is twenty-nine days, twelve hours and forty-four minutes. At the dark phase, the bright face of the moon is turned away from the earth and after a few days the crescent moon becomes visible. This crescent gradually increases until the moon is half full and visible at the zenith when the sun sets. The moon then increases in light until it reaches full and rises as the sun sets. After the full, the moon then decreases in light until the sun and the moon rise together.

Most women interact with the lunar cycle in one of two ways; their menstruation coincides either with the full moon phase or with the dark moon phase. The period of a woman's cycle may not be exactly the same as that of the moon, but it may lengthen or shorten so that menstruation fluctuates around the times of the full or dark moon each month.

Exercise

You should have looked up the relevant phases of the moon for your journal. Now start to notice also the actual phases and positioning of the moon in the sky. If possible, try to go outside and notice how the light of each different phase affects the way you feel emotionally and intuitively. Try to imagine the feminine energies for each phase; these may take on the form of ancient goddesses, of women you regard as archetypes of each phase, or of music, animals, seasons or abstract patterns.

To gain a greater understanding of the changes which occur in your creativity the energies of the four phases of menstruation and lunation need to be examined. Firstly, however, it is important that the information which you have collected each month is presented in a form which you can use to look for patterns.

THE MOON DIAL

Once you have collected information about your own cycle for a few months, it will probably become quite copious and difficult to sort through. The *Moon Dial* is a simple device which enables you to compare each month's findings and to summarize these to produce a general guide to your own menstrual cycle. The cocept of the Moon Dial has been adapted from an idea originally proposed by Penelope Shuttle and Peter Redgrove in their book *The Wise Wound*.

For the first month, start by drawing a large circle on a piece of paper. Divide the circumference into the number of days in your cycle for that month, then join the divisions with lines to the centre. Mark on the outside of the circle the calendar dates and on the inside of the circle the day number of your cycle. Write in the relevant sectors the different phases of the moon (Figure 3).

Go through the information for each day and mark next to the relevant sector the following details (if recorded) in note form:

1. *Energy level* – dynamic, sociable, low, withdrawn.
2. *Emotions* – peaceful, harmonious, angry, irritable, loving, magnanimous, motherly, intuitive, psychic.
3. *Health* – fatigue, quality of sleep, food cravings, physical changes.
4. *Sexuality* – active, passive, erotic, sensual, demanding, aggressive, none, loving, caring, lustful.
5. *Dreams* – sexual acts, interaction with men and women, occurrence of strong colours, animals, menstrual and magical content, predictive/psychic dreams and recurring dreams.

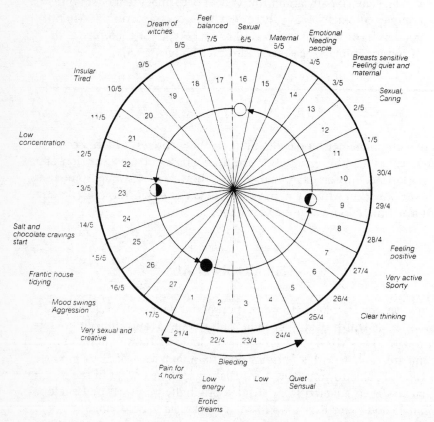

Figure 3. The Moon Dial

6.   *Outward expression* – creativity, sporting pursuits, confidence, organizational ability, concentration, ability to cope, how you dress.

This will make quite a cluttered diagram, but you may be able to simplify it by grouping similar days together. Do the same with each of the other months and you should begin to see some patterns emerging. The correspondences will not be exact, but you may find that around certain days in the month you experience similar energies or physical changes and that you have similar dream themes before menstruation or ovulation. Summarize these correspondences in a single Moon Dial. If you find it difficult to see any correspondences between the Moon Dials, continue taking notes for a few more months. You may find the section in this chapter on 'The Moon Dial and Everyday Life' will give you some guidance on what to look for.

As stated previously, the journal entries and subsequent Moon Dials are meant to be an ongoing project to keep you in touch with your cycle over the years. You will find that after a while you know your reaction to your cycle so well that you will need only to record unusual occurrences which may suggest a change in your cycle. As well as noting similarities in the timing of physical changes over the months, you will also notice recurring phases of particular emotional, creative and sexual energies.

In mythology and legend, the energies which a woman goes through each month in her menstrual cycle were seen as a four-phase rhythm which reflected the lunar phases. In the menstrual cycle the Virgin and the waxing moon represented the phase from the end of bleeding to around ovulation. The energies of this phase are similar to those of a young maiden, being generative, dynamic and inspirational. The Mother and the full moon represented the period around ovulation. The energies of motherhood and the Mother phase are also similar in the energy and ability to nourish, sustain and empower. The inner creative energies of the Mother arise to create new life.

The withdrawal of light in the darkening phase of the waning moon reflected the withdrawal of physical energy from ovulation to menstruation, and the increase in a woman's sexuality, creativity, magic, destructive inner energies and awareness. These energies are found in folklore personified as witches, enchantresses, vampires, seductresses, sorceresses and wicked stepmothers. The term 'enchantress' has been chosen for this phase in *Red Moon* because it can denote a woman of any menstrual age who has the power of magic and of her sex to create or to destroy. The image of the trapped and entombed Merlin, robbed of his magical knowledge by the beautiful and sexual enchantress Nimue, reflects the power of the

Enchantress. In the Enchantress phase, the creative energies which would have gone into making a child are released and given form in the world.

The dark moon and the black Hag represented the phase of menstruation. The Hag reflected the woman's physical energies withdrawn from the outer world and the turning in of her awareness to the inner world of the spirit. In the Hag phase of menstruation the inner creative energies are gestated in the mind to produce new life and idea children.

The waxing and waning phases are times of change and the full moon and dark moon phases are times of pivot. Within a woman the changing phases are those of the Virgin and Enchantress and the pivot phases are those of the Mother and the Hag. The Virgin phase is an ascent into the light, manifest outward aspect of a woman's nature and the Enchantress phase is a descent from the outward nature into the dark, unmanifest, inner aspect. The Mother phase balances the outward expression of energy with the inner expression of love and the Hag phase balances the stillness of the inner world with the gestation of a new cycle (Figure 4). Although the diagram is drawn with equal parts, on a particular Moon Dial for an individual woman the phases may look more like Figure 5.

Although the cycle is divided into four phases, the demarcation between these phases is not rigid; rather, each phase merges naturally into the next in the flow of energies in the menstrual cycle. This idea found expression in folk stories in the magical transformations of women into animals, of old women into maidens, maidens into women and women into vampires. The four-fold lunar rhythm is the simplest image of the menstrual cycle, but some women may find that their own cycle expresses itself in a more complicated pattern.

The Virgin Energies

The Virgin energies are dynamic and radiating. The Virgin phase is a time when each woman is free from the procreative cycle and belongs only to herself. The woman becomes self-confident, sociable and able to cope with all the mundane aggravations of life. She experiences greater determination, ambition and concentration and she can achieve more in her work. It is a time to start new projects. Her sexuality is new and fresh and this phase becomes a time of fun

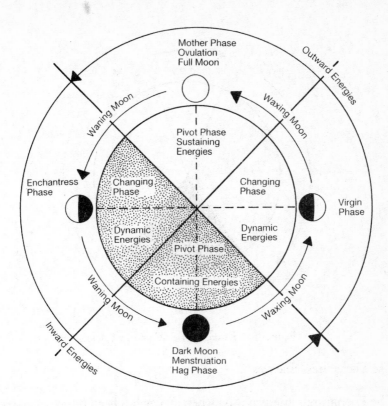

Figure 4. The White Moon Cycle

and joy. Her whole outlook expresses enthusiasm for the outer world and for experiencing it to the full!

The Mother Energies

The Mother energies appear around the time of ovulation and are also radiating, but on a different frequency to those from the Virgin. The Mother phase is a time when women lose their sense of self in preparedness for the selflessness of motherhood. The woman's own wants and needs become less important to her; she becomes caring, radiating love and harmony. Her sexuality blossoms into an experience of deep love and sharing. The woman is able to take on responsibilities, to nourish and give birth to new projects and ideas and to sustain those already in existence. She may find that she becomes a magnet to people and that people will turn to her for help and support.

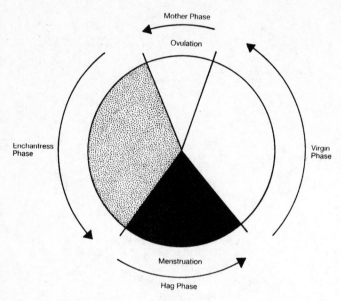

Figure 5.   Example of a Woman's Cycle

The Enchantress Energies

The Enchantress energies arise when an egg has been released, but not fertilized. The woman starts to experience the inner side of her nature. She becomes aware of the mysteries underlying nature and her sexuality becomes powerful. She becomes aware also of her own personal magic and power and the effect it can have on men. The energies can become fiery and when released can manifest in tremendous, unrestrained creativity. As the phase of the Hag approaches, the woman may become intolerant of the mundane world and her concentration decreases but her intuition and dream capacity increase.

The Hag Energies

The Hag energies are experienced at menstruation as a deepening of the inner awareness of the Enchantress phase. The energies become containing and intuitive, no longer seeking outward expression except in the occasional burst of ecstatic vision. The woman interacts more with her dreams; she feels part of nature and intuitively recognizes the patterns underlying it.

The Hag phase is a time of introspection, a time to step away from the mundane world, to sleep and dream, to express magic gently and to slow one's life down. It is a time to seek answers to problems and to learn to accept the past and the uncertainty of the future. The woman becomes open to the older, more primal energies and instincts. Her sexuality blossoms as at the full moon, but rather than bringing her energies into the physical world, it heightens her spirituality.

At any one time, a woman holds part of the dark and light energies within herself. There are no fixed divisions between each phase; each is a gradual flow from one energy to another. As the Virgin and Enchantress, she contains both light and dark in changing amounts and as the Mother and Hag, she holds the seed of menstruation and ovulation within herself. With the release of the egg in the Mother phase, the process towards menstruation begins and with the release of the womb lining in the Hag phase the ripening of the next egg for ovulation starts. The seed of light within darkness and the seed of darkness within light can be seen in the yin yang diagram as a flow of energies from one to the other (Figure 6).

You may find that in your own cycle you can subdivide the energies further. By identifying each phase within yourself and giving it some type of symbol that you can relate to, you are able to start accepting and reawakening all sides of your nature.

Women's menstruation tends to occur around the time of the full moon or dark moon. Ovulation with the full moon corresponds to the White Moon cycle, which is celebrated in most fertility religions and

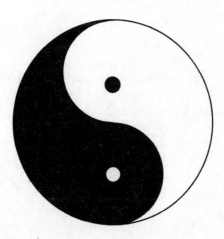

Figure 6. Yin Yang Symbol

rites. The fertile power of the woman and the full moon coincide, providing the best conditions for the woman to express her creative energies in conception. The White Moon cycle became the cycle of the 'good mother', the only aspect of womanhood acceptable to the patriarchal society.

Less acceptable was the cycle which resulted from ovulation at the time of the dark moon. As the full moon rises through the thicker atmosphere at the horizon, it is often stained blood red; the Red Moon cycle occurs when menstruation coincides with the full moon. The personal cycle of the woman still passes through the phases of Virgin, Mother, Enchantress and Hag, but these are 180° out of phase to those of the moon (Figure 7). Ovulation occurs in the darkness of the moon, with the creative energies being released in the increasing light of the moon.

The Red Moon cycle shows an orientation away from the expression of the energies in procreation and the material world and towards inner development and its expression. As this cycle was seen by men as more powerful and less controllable, it became the cycle of the 'evil woman', the seductress, the wise woman or the ugly witch, whose sexuality was applied to something other than the formation of the next generation.

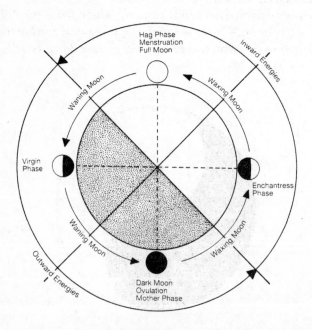

Figure 7.   The Red Moon Cycle

Those women who lived in rhythm with the Red Moon cycle would have been closeted away from the full moon rites and celebrations of the ovulating women. They were the reminder of the dark half of the bright full moon.

Both cycles are expressions of the feminine energies and neither is more powerful or more correct than the other. You may find that through your life your cycles will change orientation between the Red and White Moon cycles depending on your circumstances, ambitions, emotions and goals.

Exercise

Look at your summary Moon Dial and note where in your cycle the different energies seem to occur. You may find that to start with, you are aware only of experiencing some of the energies for some of the time. The energies are still within you, but external influences such as stress and exhaustion as well as a breakdown in the intuitive link between your body and your mind may make it difficult for you to become aware of them. Use four coloured pencils to colour in the days on which you are aware of the different energies. Over the months, as you become increasingly aware of your cycle, you will be able to produce a coloured Moon Dial which will become the key to your menstrual cycle.

TOWARDS SELF AWARENESS

Bleeding is one of the most taboo subjects in modern society and if a woman shows that she is bleeding it can be very embarrassing. It is worth examining your own reaction to your monthly blood to discover why you feel the way you do. How do you feel about your blood staining your clothes? Are you able to touch your blood? How do you feel if your partner sees your blood? Do you wear tampons and expect to live life in the same way as the rest of the month? Are you aware of the menstruation of other women with whom you come into contact and do you know their cycles?

The question may be posed: how many women are truly conscious of their bleeding as something other than a monthly function which is annoying, messy and gets in the way of life? Nowadays, a large percentage of the female population use some form of tampon every month, enabling a woman at her time of bleeding to lead a 'normal active' life, without having to worry about stains and unsightly bumps on her clothes and allowing her to take part in swimming, exercise and other physical activities. The tampon has given a freedom of movement not available with the sanitary towel, but it also lessens awareness of the actual act of bleeding. Unless you are forced into an awareness of your cycle through premenstrual syndrome or period pains, you can become totally detached from your bleeding, being unaware of it until you have to change a tampon.

The social stigma attached to women's bleeding is that it is *uncontrollable*. If a woman is bleeding freely, she is aware that she cannot stop it from happening; it is as inevitable as the energies associated with menstruation. What should be a natural symbol of the beauty of the female cycle has become a stigma reminding society of the uncontrollable and unrestrained nature of women, which has been viewed as inferior and degrading. The use of tampons mentally blocks the evidence of the woman's menstruation and, indeed, her own acceptance of her menstruation.

This is not to suggest that tampons should not be used if desired; but allocating a time when they are not used allows a woman to become aware of the sensations of her bleeding, giving her an opportunity to accept it and to bring that awareness into her everyday life.

Exercise

If you wear tampons, allow yourself some time during your menstruation to experience your bleeding. Use sanitary towels or make your own from cloth or tissues and cotton wool. This gives you the opportunity to use recyclable and unbleached products if you wish. You may find that for practical reasons you can only do this when you are not actually working or rushing around, as the effect of experiencing bleeding becomes very noticeable in the way you move, behave and perform the tasks which you want to do. Note your experiences in your journal and compare them with the later section 'The Moon Dial and Everyday Life'.

Inner Awareness

The Moon Dial is a record of the outer expression of your monthly cycle in terms of emotions, health, sexuality and creativity. Having begun to learn about your cycle's outer form, it is also necessary to learn its inner form if you are to begin interacting with its energies. A woman's menstrual cycle can be sensitive to many factors including extreme weight loss, drugs, illness and anxiety, shock or stress. Often a woman may experience some change in her cycle such as late bleeding, altered flow or increased pain or discomfort if she is under stress. In this situation, the womb and the menstrual cycle are reacting to the person's mental state. The cycle may also change its orientation with the moon, depending on the way a woman feels about her life and what she wants to achieve from it.

Conversely, depending on the hormones released during the different stages of the cycle, the menstrual cycle can have a dramatic effect on the woman's physical abilities, her personality, her creative and sexual energies. The link between the woman and her womb is two-way and she can consciously interact with this link through her subconscious. You may also cause distortion in this link and therefore distress in your cycle, either by hating the effects of your cycle on your body or by restricting the flow and expression of your cycle's energies and your body's needs. This distress causes more distortion of your link with your cycle, causing a self-sustaining feedback loop. To break this loop and recreate a positive link, you must become aware of your womb at an inner level, learn its cycle and energies and learn to accept your own cyclic nature.

The easiest way to establish a link with your menstrual cycle is to use imagination, visualization and thoughts to become aware of the womb and to influence it. It often does not occur to women that they carry a womb at all, except at menstruation or pregnancy. The following exercises are designed to awaken awareness of your womb and to open up an inner relationship between it and the conscious mind. Once these exercises are experienced, a conscious link will be established enabling the use of visualization to ease the womb through difficult times in the cycle, to renew your link with your cycle when you feel distant from it and for the subconscious to open up the meaning of menstruation for you.

You may find that it is easier to do the following visualizations if they are read onto audio tape and played back. Make sure that when you make the tape you read slowly, allowing yourself time to build the scenario in your mind and to interact with the scene.

Exercise

This exercise is designed to establish a conscious link between
your mind and your womb. Once you have made that link, it
can be reawakened at any time during the day or during the cycle.
By recognizing that the mind is linked to the womb and reacts
to changes in the womb and that the womb will react in turn
to mental changes, the link becomes a tool whereby symptoms
such as an irregular cycle, period pains or premenstrual tension
can be accepted and integrated into your life.

Use the following exercise at any time during the month to
re-establish your awareness of your womb. It does not have to
be done in a quiet room with candles every time, although it
does help to make the first encounter special. Your womb is
with you all the time, so acknowledge it whilst working, doing
the shopping, whatever!

Awareness Of Your Womb

Sit in a quiet room in a comfortable position. You may already
have experience of visualization; if not, either sit in an upright
chair with your hands resting in your lap or on your thighs
and your head tipped slightly forward, or lie on the floor with
your arms and legs slightly spread out with your head resting on
something soft. (The danger with this position is that you may
have a tendency to fall asleep.)

Start by closing your eyes and relaxing your body. As you
breathe out, imagine all the tensions and worries of the everyday
world washing out of your body into the earth beneath your feet.
Be aware of your feet and the feeling of pressure on them. Allow
your awareness to travel up your body, acknowledging your feet
and legs, your arms and hands, your abdomen and chest, your
face and shoulders, and the rhythm of your breathing. Finally,
become aware of your body as a whole.

Then bring your awareness down towards your womb. See in
your mind the central womb with the fallopian tubes on either
side and the ovaries on the ends. Become aware of first one
ovary and then the other. You may find that you begin to
experience a feeling of tightness or of warmth growing in the
area of your womb. Now visualize your womb slowly enlarging,
until it envelops your body. Feel the fallopian tubes reaching

out from your shoulders and visualize your arms stretching out like the branches, holding the cluster of eggs like fruit in your hands. Allow the creative energy of your womb to rise up inside you, along your arms and into your fingers, making them tingle. Feel completely at one with the image of your womb.

Gradually lower your arms and slowly allow the image of your womb to shrink back to its normal size. Mentally acknowledge its presence and then become aware of the rest of your body. Finally open your eyes and take a deep breath.

You may feel very peaceful after the exercise or you may feel the need to use the energy raised to create something. You do not have to go out and create a masterpiece; use the energy in your everyday life, in crafts, music, poetry, in cooking, sewing, gardening or in your relationships with other people, helping them to heal or to solve problems.

The Womb Tree

The first part of this exercise introduces you to the image of the Womb Tree. You can then use this image at any time to interact with your womb and menstrual cycle on an inner level. The second part of the exercise introduces you to your Guardian, who holds the key to the creative forces which arise in your body and mind and who can help you to rebalance any problems and to open up the inner knowledge of your menstrual cycle. The Guardian may take any form and may surprise you in the image it presents. You may also find that the scene in the visualizations will take on its own form to suit the particular time of the month.

Both exercises can be used at any time of the month to interact with your womb or to learn of your inner nature. You may wish to keep a record of any insights which you gain.

Establishing The Link

Relax in the same way as for the first exercise. Become aware that you are standing surrounded by a silvery mist. As the mist gradually parts, you walk into a moonlit glade. In the centre of the glade stands a huge tree on a mound rising from the middle of a circular pool. As you approach, you see that the trunk is silvery-pink and it splits into two branches, each ending in clusters of leaves and numerous shining red fruit. Above the tree, appearing to brush the top leaves, you see a full moon flooding the scene with silver light.

You feel very still and calm, filled with an air of wonder. The whole tree seems to shimmer with life and you feel an inner link with it. You walk to the edge of the pool just within arm's length of the leaves, which reach out over the water towards you. The water is dark blue and you can see the roots of the tree disappearing into the depths. Something stirs in your mind and you become aware of small tendrils, like roots, linking your mind to your womb. You feel that the water is alive and looking into it you see your own reflection with the moon's light dancing above. The water holds within its depths the mysteries of the universe and you recognize the universal link between woman and the moon, the womb and the moon's cycle, the womb and the mind, and the mind and the womb.

Stay for a while, feeling the closeness of the tree. When you are ready to leave, allow the mists to once more cover the scene and gradually become aware of your body. Before you open your eyes feel the tendrils in your mind which link it to the womb in your belly.

Meeting The Guardian

Relax as before and visualize yourself standing on warm grass in the sunshine. Stand for a while noticing the feel of the grass on your bare feet, the scent in the air, the quality of the sunlight and the season of the year. In front of you stands your Womb Tree and as you walk towards the tree you notice that the season has touched its branches. A light breeze rustles the leaves and looking up into the branches you ask for your Guardian to appear. As you lower your eyes, you find your Guardian standing in front of you. Notice all you can about the Guardian's appearance.

You feel a subtle aura of power as the Guardian silently holds out an object. You see that the object is a beautiful miniature building shaped like a short cross with a dome in the centre, made from gold with intricate patterns and studded with gems. You are amazed by its beauty and craftsmanship and as the Guardian lifts the dome you see that it is a box containing a chalice. The chalice is made of gold on the outside and silver on the inside and fits snugly into the box. Inside the chalice you see a small amount of dark red liquid which nearly covers a ring inset with a huge rectangular-cut ruby.

The Guardian lifts the chalice from the box and offers it to you, telling you that if you were to touch the ring, the wine would poison you but if you drink the wine first, you may retrieve the ring safely. You lift the chalice to your lips and drink the wine, tasting the heavy scents of spices on your tongue. As you lift the ring from the chalice and place it on your finger, you feel that something important has just happened. You feel a warmth in your womb and an inner strength giving you confidence and insight. You are Woman and are all that being a woman means. You accept your body and trust in your nature, knowing that you are as much a part of the inner world as of the outer world.

With that acceptance and trust comes a feeling of grace and as you become aware of your real body, you carry that grace and measured strength into it.

Contact with your Guardian can be made at any future time through visualization of your Womb Tree.

A woman's inner awareness of her menstrual cycle may also be found in the appearance of Moon Animals in her dreams and imagination. You may have found in your Moon Dial records that you dream of certain animals during the month; they may herald your ovulation or bleeding, or reflect hidden fears and trauma. These animals offer understanding of your true nature, bringing to your conscious mind guidance which may normally be repressed. Keeping a dream record is important, as it brings the awareness of the animals and their wisdom into your waking mind. The relationship with the Moon Animals is not restricted to passive or reactive dreaming; they can be brought into the conscious mind by daydreaming, visualization, meditation or by writing stories or poems about them or painting them.

Repression and restriction of your nature can result in the Moon Animals exhibiting nightmarish qualities, but only because they reflect the fear and dislike you feel for your own cycle and therefore for yourself. Your subconscious will make use of the animal image to express the information in a form which the conscious mind will understand.

Exercise

If you have not found any particular animals in your dreams or if you want to stage a setting in order to meet a particular Moon

Animal, you may use the description of the meeting of Eve and the Moon Animals in *The Awakening* as a basis for your own visualization.

As you become aware of the animals, the one which has particular importance for you will step forward to meet you. The animal may speak to you, show you scenes, offer you an object of significance or offer you emotions. If you have had a dream about a particular animal, ask it to come forward and ask for help in interpreting its meaning. It may be that you will have to relive the dream again before the meaning becomes clear.

You may like to try the visualization before going to sleep, allowing the animal the freedom of your dreams to help you.

USING YOUR AWARENESS

Now that you have used visualizations to establish an inner link with your womb, you may also use the images at any time during your cycle to realign yourself with the cycle or to aid yourself through times of menstrual distress.

If you suffer from pain at any stage during your cycle, you can use the image of the Womb Tree as a way of interacting with your womb and easing the discomfort, as follows.

Exercise

Find yourself a relatively comfortable position in which to sit or lie. If possible, try to sit or kneel upright. Take a deep breath and as you breathe out relax any muscle tension which may have occurred in reaction to the pain. Do not concentrate on the pain at this time, but be aware of your womb in the same way as you did in the Womb Awareness exercise and allow a feeling of warmth to build. Visualize your Womb Tree over your womb and send it thoughts of love and caring. This reinforces the link of acceptance between your mind and your womb.

Accept the pain and do not attempt to fight against it. After a few minutes, visualize a cascade of warm water flowing over your body from head to toe. Breathe slowly and deeply and as you breathe out allow the warmth to carry away the pain and to ease any muscle spasms.

Although this exercise may not remove the discomfort completely, it can help you to get through the worst moments. Dealing with pain is not easy; it takes practice and it requires you to remain calm both mentally and physically. Most importantly, do not fight the pain. Allow it to happen, but ease your way through it with love and acceptance.

If you suffer badly from menstrual distress, either mentally or physically, use the Womb Awareness and Womb Tree exercises throughout the month to maintain a constant, positive link with your cycle. You may also need to review your lifestyle to see if you are repressing your cyclic nature or energies. The different phases of the menstrual cycle and different ways to interact with them will be considered later in this chapter.

To realign your cycle with your mind or with the moon's phases, go outside into the light of the full moon. Stand where you can see the moon and be aware of its light in the sky and in your mind. Feel the presence of your womb and become aware of your Womb Tree. See the full moon resting in the branches of your womb tree, reflecting its light in the surrounding water. Feel the tendrils of the tree roots deep in the water of your mind. Be aware of the moon in your womb, the moon in your mind and the moon in the sky. You may like to view this as a rededication each month of your conscious nature to your deeper cyclic nature. It makes no difference to this exercise if your personal phase does not match that of the moon.

If you are trying to align your cycle with the moon's phases, sleep in view of the full moon or, if this is not possible, sleep with a light on during the time of the full moon. Remember, though, that you do not have to have the same rhythm as the moon to be in harmony with the phases and energies of your own cycle.

After your phase of bleeding, you may feel that you wish to mark the end of one cycle and the beginning of the new one; the end of the dark phase and the beginning of the Virgin phase. In ancient Athens, women at the end of their bleeding would visit the temple of Athene to wash their bloodied laundry and to be reborn as virgins. The following exercise may be used as a cleansing after menstruation, a washing away of the old in preparation for the new, or as a purification and rededication of your womb and cycle if you have suffered intrusion or abuse.

Exercise: Cleansing

The cleansing exercise is based on intent. You can include as much symbolism as you have the time or the need for and the only practical requirement is some water. A bath is the most luxurious way of performing the cleansing, but you may use a shower or a simple basin of water if you prefer.

If you are taking a bath, allow yourself to relax in the water, removing yourself from the worries and tensions of the day. After a little while, picture the moon's phase in the sky and feel yourself bathing in its light or darkness. Be aware of the water surrounding you, of the water of your body and the pull of the moon's tide on it. Feel the presence of your womb and visualize your Womb Tree with each of the moon's phases resting in its branches. Cup some water in your hands, raise them and as the water trickles between your fingers feel the light or darkness of the moon flowing down your body from your head to your womb. Keep your hands raised for as long as you feel the need and then gradually lower them, allowing yourself to feel cleansed, renewed, pure and at peace.

Enjoy this feeling for as long as you can and then leave the water. As the water droplets drip from you and the bath empties, feel the old cycle with all its emotions and problems flowing away with the water, allowing you to emerge like Aphrodite, new and beautiful.

THE MOON DIAL AND EVERYDAY LIFE

Women have been very much restricted by society to the masculine, linear view of the personality. The formation of the Moon Dial from a woman's own experiences over several months not only emphasizes the cyclic nature of her personality, but also enables her to grasp the concept intellectually and to feel for herself the truth and validity of the rhythms of her life. Since the natural expression of her cyclic nature has been repressed by society, it is necessary for each woman to relearn this expression from her own cycle.

The following sections look in more detail at the four major phases of the menstrual cycle, suggesting different ways in which these phases express themselves and how a woman can interact with them. As previously considered, the four-fold division is only the simplest division of the cycle and each woman's cycle will manifest in its own form but the ideas and concepts may be used as a guide to general interpretation and interaction.

Each section suggests an awareness exercise designed to provide a less intellectual and more experiential approach to the energies. If possible, these exercises should be performed during the appropriate phase in the cycle, although they can be used at any time to rebalance the energies within the cycle. As with the previous visualizations, the exercises may be easier to do if you record the words onto audio tape. Each section will also consider the imbalance caused when a woman allows one phase of energies to dominate her life and a list of keywords are given which may be used later in the section 'Expansion of the Moon Dial'.

The Hag Phase

The Hag phase is a time of withdrawal, a time to listen to your inner self and body. The phase may start at menstruation or slightly before it and ends at around the time when bleeding stops. There are no rigid boundaries between the different phases; the energies flow freely from one phase to the other and you will gradually become aware of the change in the energies which mark the beginning of the next phase. The Hag phase is a time of pivot; it balances the inward expression of the intuitive energies with the outward expression of the intellect.

The time of bleeding is a time when the barriers between the conscious and subconscious mind are lowered, enabling you to open up your awareness and interact with your body consciousness. Although withdrawn, the phase is not negative; there is often a sense of acceptance and of being part of everything and this is an opportunity for you to allow your inner self expression in your waking mind. The creative energies are no longer inspirational, but appear visionary through the ability to see patterns and gain knowledge. The phase of the Hag is a time of stillness and gestation, before you once more break into the world in the white light of the new moon crescent. It is the pivot point between the end of one cycle and the beginning of the new one.

With menstruation, the slowing down process of the Enchantress phase is completed. The body has less physical energy, it may be heavy with swollen breasts and belly and generally needs more sleep. The mundane world becomes less important; attention to small details and everyday needs become annoying and impossible to concentrate on. The need to withdraw is the need for a woman to become aware of her own inner levels. Socializing and even speech can become unnecessary. The inner and outer worlds can become mixed, the stillness and the need to dream remaining with the woman as she goes about everyday tasks. This can often feel like living in two worlds at the same time.

Mental processes also slow down and may even stop altogether at a point of meditation or a trancelike reverie. Emotions, however, well easily to the surface and the extreme sensitivity of empathy can make the mundane world too much to bear. Sexual energies aroused at this phase can reach a depth of experience not found during the rest of the cycle. There may be the need to express deep feelings of love and romance and the need to see this expressed in return by the partner. Sex at this time can be an expression of this intense, almost spiritual, love between two people.

INTERACTING WITH THE HAG ENERGIES

The simplest way of reflecting inner feelings in an outward form is through your appearance. Clothes are a creative expression of your inner self and of your reaction to your body and the world around you. In choosing clothes, hairstyle, make-up and jewellery, you are reflecting your feelings and expressing them in the form of image, colour and shape. This is a process which women go through every day, but because it is mostly carried out almost subconsciously, it is not viewed as a creative expression. By consciously choosing clothes and colours to match your phases, you are awakening within your everyday consciousness an awareness of the link between yourself, your body and your cycle.

Altering your clothes throughout your cycle reinforces the qualities of each phase within you. Being aware of your phase and dressing to express it subtly alters the way you walk, your mannerisms and gestures and your attitude towards people, because it is constantly reinforcing the nature of the phase within you. You may also find that men and women will react to you differently at each phase by picking up this expression on a subconscious level.

During the Hag phase, you may feel drawn towards the wearing of comforting or comfortable clothes. These may be old 'faithful' clothes which are easy to wear or free-flowing clothes like skirts or dresses. You may find that your breasts and belly are large at this time, so choose clothes which accept the roundness of your figure. If you are very shape-conscious you may choose to dress to cover your roundness, but do not fight your body or regard it with hatred; with the acceptance of the swelling of the body comes a serenity and a confidence in its fuller shape. Like the prehistoric Venus figurines, the fuller body is to be honoured.

Choose colours which you feel are appropriate. You may wish to wear red to show your bleeding, black to indicate your withdrawal or perhaps purple to express a more esoteric nature. You may find that a shawl or wrap becomes a symbol of your withdrawal, a protective barrier between yourself and the world.

The Hag phase also brings a need for quiet and a need to be still. Most women's lives are so hectic that they do not allow themselves to menstruate naturally. The body loses blood, but the tampon reduces the woman's awareness of this and she carries on as 'normal', perhaps needing to push herself even harder both mentally and physically in order to achieve her usual working expectations. In many cases, a woman may wonder why she is so tired and unable to work, only to *remember* that she is menstruating.

Everyday life does not stop for the menstruating woman, but in today's society more than ever there is less and less time for women to withdraw, with the expectations and demands of running a household and working for a living. It is difficult for women to accept the menstruating side of their nature if they are not allowed time to stop and listen to it. The modern woman has to find a balance, to meet her work requirements, her family's needs and at the same time to meet her own needs. One way of meeting your needs at menstruation is to allow yourself to menstruate both *mentally* and *physically* when you can. Ideally this should occur every month but even if you do not have the time every month, it is still worth making the attempt when you can.

The physical need at menstruation is to slow your pace of life. If you can, try to spend some time away from the demands of work, family or partners, doing what you feel you need to do, even if only for an hour in the evening. Explain to family or partner that nothing is wrong but that you need some quiet time, on your own if necessary, to slow down and rest. Once you start to *allow* yourself to slow down, you will find that this process comes naturally and will alter the comparative urgency and priorities of things you have to do. Try not to take on too much at this time; arrange your day to suit the way you feel at menstruation. If you have to maintain your pace within the world during the day, it is even more important to allow yourself time to interact with your menstruation in the evenings. Try to let go of all those things which demand your time but which are not really essential; you may find that your normal tendency is not to bother with these things at this time anyway.

By only doing what is essential, you will feel able to cope and less under the pressure of everyday expectations. If you find that you don't have the energy to work as hard or as fast during the Hag phase, try to organize your life so that you can use the dynamic energy of the Virgin phase to catch up. Obviously, it is not possible to arrange this every month, but whenever it is possible it will bring greater satisfaction to your life.

The physical slowing down can alter not only the organization of your life, but also the interaction which you have with your body. If you allow yourself to bleed, especially without using a tampon, movement and walking become slow and almost dreamlike. If you move with the slowness, your movements will become graceful, almost like dance, but if you fight against it and force movement, you may become cumbersome and unco-ordinated. Sports can become difficult at this time and you may find that you are unable to reach the levels of fitness, stamina and strength which you expect at other times of the month.

Menstruation is the time to express your conscious link with your body and the link between your body and the natural world. When bleeding, allow yourself the luxury of bathing or washing more often, not because menstruation is dirty (although hygiene is important) but because it is a way of pampering your body and of feeling well and at one with it. Use the water to wash away the old month, the feelings, problems and desires, and feel your link with the water; see it as your emotions, the water of your body which gives you life, your intuition, the fertilizing rain and the waters of your birth. Use this time to enjoy your body; use candles to bathe by and natural oils or herb extracts as scents. You may feel that you do not want to wear or use manmade products or scents. Use massage to become aware of your body, spending time on areas which usually get ignored. Often ill health can be a loss of well-being; by reconnecting with your body, with your nature and spirit, the sense of connectedness and well-being can be re-established.

You may find that you are drawn to simpler foods, such as vegetables, cereals and fruit, rather than fast food or junk foods. Your body may give you cravings for foods which you normally do not eat or sometimes you may not feel the need to eat at all. The body seems to lean towards a more natural expression at menstruation, a reflection of the need at this time to live at a simpler level.

During this time the mind, emotions and mental processes change. A woman can be slower in her thought processes and these processes may be chaotic, illogical and intuitive. You may also feel unwilling to talk or to make the effort of social contact. The ability to concentrate for long periods of time can be diminished, leading to frustration and tears.

As previously considered, the ability to cope with everyday things can be helped by reorganizing your environment or by changing your lifestyle at this time, but you may also find problems in coping emotionally. The ability to empathize with other people is greatly increased at this time and in some women this may reach almost unbearable levels, creating periods of tearfulness and emotion. You are at your most sensitive to disasters and tragedy, whether on the news or in a film or book, often living the emotions of grief of families or victims.

Crying results in the flow of emotional energies which can become part of the healing during menstruation. The emotions of grief are also a reflection of the awareness of death, of the end of the old cycle and of loss, all of which are a part of the monthly link between the woman and the rhythms of life. Although this awareness can be healing, the barrage of news of disasters from all over the world can mean that this sensitivity becomes destructive, leading to feelings of hopelessness.

You cannot carry all the grief and emotions for the whole world and so you need to protect yourself. The easiest way to do this is to isolate yourself from the television, the radio and the newspapers so that you can limit your feelings to the immediate problems of your family or friends. To isolate yourself completely from tragedy may not allow you to experience the realization of death and renewal which comes at menstruation and so a balance needs to be formed. The other way to approach these feelings is to alter your perception. Rather than passively empathizing with people, feeling their emotions as your own, you can instead practise actively feeling compassion for the people involved. By feeling *for* others, rather than *with* others, you will then be in a position to offer help. Turning empathy into compassion, you can offer help from a position of understanding.

In the Hag phase, not only does the body need more sleep, the mind also needs more time to dream. Descending into yourself, you have access to the workings of your inner life and your dreams can teach you about your body and mind.

Dreaming is not necessarily restricted to the images produced during sleep; it also includes daydreaming, fantasies and visualization, methods of dreaming whereby the conscious mind supplies a context through which the subconscious can interact. This interaction may be in the form of emotions, ideas, images or awareness. By taking time to dream, you have the capacity for vision, imaginative wisdom, foresight, insight and mystical experience.

Keep notes of your dreams and insights at this time. You may find that they alter your perception of life or offer help and understanding. They can also be used as the subject of visualization and meditation.

Prayer, magic and divination may also be used to express your inner awareness at the time of the Hag. There are many books available covering a wide range of traditions, methods of divination and expressions of prayer. If you are not already familiar with any of these, you may like to try several of the different forms to see which suits you best. You will find that in nearly all cases they give you a form in which you can actively use your ability to see patterns, to make vast leaps of insight and to use your intuition, as well as offering a method of interacting with the concept of the existence of two worlds.

The dark phase is a time to allow your emotions and intuition to flow, but it is also a time to carry out an assessment on a mental level. The death carried by the dark phase is expressed in menstruation in the death of the old month, the death of ties, emotions and behaviour which have built up over the past month which need to be released before starting anew with the waxing moon. Use this time to assess your life, your health and your relationships and to accept that events and emotions have passed, that although they were once a part of you they are no longer. You may find that you feel a deep sense of loss or emptiness. The Enchantress phase will have cut the threads which held you to the old way of life, enabling the Hag phase to give you the choice of fibres to weave into the pattern of your future life. It is a time to accept the changes in life and to celebrate the continuing cycle which is yourself.

The Hag phase brings a yearning for connection with nature, the creative energies and the intuitive inner self. The creative energies are at this time unstructured, reacting to stimuli and creating ideas which can either be developed mentally or discarded. The Hag woman can be very sensitive to archetypal images, whether they appear in books, art, television or music, and these archetypes can stimulate further images and expression.

Try to actively stimulate your mind by looking at artwork and sculpture, reading folk stories and legends (children's books are the best, as they contain illustrations which can help to stimulate ideas) or by watching theatre. You will find that certain images will call to you on an inner level. The ideas stimulated will need expression within the Hag phase, as the power of the imagery fades with the Virgin phase. Your mind will often pick up archetypal images from the world around you, sometimes without you being consciously aware of it.

The Hag phase is the end of the outwardly dynamic, creative energies of the cycle. This ending can bring a sense of loss if the new, inner quality is not recognized, but it also provides an opportunity to cut the ties which hold you to work, ideas and other forms which you have already created, enabling the seeds of new ideas to grow in the dark womb of menstruation.

There are some differences in the emphasis of the Hag energies depending on whether you are bleeding with the full moon or the dark moon. A woman with the White Moon cycle, bleeding with the dark moon, becomes linked to the deepest levels of her awareness, reminding her that there exists more than just the manifest world. A woman with a Red Moon cycle, bleeding with the full moon, brings the energies and mysteries of the inner darkness out into the manifest world.

Sometimes, certain phases of a woman's cycle can become repressed and others allowed to dominate. If a woman allows the Hag phase of her nature to dominate, she can develop a tendency to live in her own mind, in dreams or fantasies, with no real grip on the ordinary world. She can be someone who withdraws from the world and its events, often isolating herself from other people and living alone. A woman who represses the Hag energies represses the inner strength and wisdom which she holds within herself and stifles her ability to grow through change.

Exercise: Menstrual Meditation

Sit or lie somewhere quiet and dark and allow your eyes to become accustomed to the darkness. Feel safe and secure, cushioned by the comforting, supporting warmth of the darkness. In it you feel the ability and luxury to forget. Feel around you the darkness which lies within all things and the inner darkness of yourself. Open yourself to it; there is no fear, just acceptance, love and healing. Above you, you see the darkness of space and the shimmer of galaxies and stars. You see the dark moon and feel the presence of the light behind it. Feel the acceptance of darkness within yourself, not as evil but as a source of renewal and transformation. Darkness is the source of all being, the potential in the womb, the darkness from which you were born and the darkness to which you will return.

KEYWORDS

Darkness / Hecate / seed / Persephone / womb / winter / oneness / potential / earth / cave / torch / tomb / snake / owl / universe / dark moon / vision / prophecy / wisdom / patterns / renewal / gestation.

The Virgin Phase

The Virgin phase is a time of expressing the inner energies and of bringing the subconscious into the light of day. It is the time to take hold of the insights and ideas gained in the darkness of the Crone phase and give them expression in the everyday world. The Virgin woman has the opportunity to regenerate her life. The grieving time for the past month is over, the woman has 'touched base' with her inner self through her menstruation and she has renewed the strength and confidence which come from her inner self.

The phase of the Virgin is a time of rebirth, of new energy and enthusiasm. With menstruation over, the body has become slimmer, more energetic, lithe and 'younger' and the destructive energies and trancelike slowness become dynamic and focused towards new goals. The joy of life becomes expressed through the newness of the body in the beginning of a new cycle and through the body's interaction with the world around it. The body becomes important as a way of expressing and reflecting life and has more physical stamina and energy, requiring less sleep. You regain self-confidence in both your body and your abilities.

In the menstrual phase, most women experience emotions and their sexuality at a deep, inner level. In the Virgin phase, however, you become outgoing, funloving and flirtatious. Like a young maiden, your sexual nature is bright and new. The self-confidence in your body adds a young sensuality to the way you behave, making sexual acts full of fun and love. The first sexual act after bleeding renews the bond between each woman and her partner, mimicking her first encounter.

The Maiden phase is one of mental as well as physical dynamism. You become mentally strong, analytical and clear thinking. You develop an ability to see structure, to itemize and prioritize, to begin new projects and to retain the enthusiasm to get them started against the odds. You also become more independent, requiring less support, comfort and encouragement from others and with the inner drive to push through things you believe in against any opposition. To some men, this determined, sharp-thinking, strong woman can seem threatening.

You will also attain the strength to stand up and protect those who you feel are weaker or suffering from injustice. The Virgin is the active side of your inner nature; what you feel deeply or intuitively becomes the basis for determined action. The creative energies appear in sudden mental leaps of bright inspiration which, with the enhanced abilities of strong concentration and attention to detail, enable you to achieve the goals you have set for yourself.

The Virgin phase is also a phase of communication and sociability. You may well find that you develop a need to meet people, to get out and about and to have fun! This phase may begin as soon as bleeding stops or during the days of final blood. It is a phase of constant change, with the energies radiating and flowing towards the Mother phase.

INTERACTING WITH THE VIRGIN ENERGIES

During the Virgin phase you may find that you wish to wear a younger style of clothes and brighter colours. As your body is feeling slimmer and more athletic, you may want to show it off in tighter fitting and more sensual styles, but with overtones of fun rather than overt seduction. After the flowing skirts of menstruation, the freedom of trousers or jeans suits this phase of activity and energy. Have fun with your clothes, wear white if you feel like it and 'sexy virgin' underwear with plenty of frilly white lace! Your sexuality is new and funloving, so express it in your hairstyle, clothes, jewellery and activities. As the phase progresses, you may find that the young, frivolous energy gradually matures and deepens, but that you still retain the feeling of independence and the need for activity. You may want to show this gradual change in the way you dress.

The Virgin phase is a phase of activity, both mental and physical. Try to find time to take some exercise, even if it is only walking instead of using the car. The pleasure you take in your body and the world around you becomes an expression of the pleasure of life itself. If you have time, learn a new sport, take up an old one again or learn dance or aerobics. If you can do these with a group of friends it can be more fun and will also meet your need to be more sociable. With the increase in self-confidence and physical energy, this phase is a good time to start a diet to lose weight or to take up a healthy eating and exercise routine. (During the month the body's flexibility, stamina and strength will change constantly. Do not let this put you off attempting a sport or physical exercise. It is better to do some exercise when you are able and rest when you are not, rather than do nothing because you feel that you cannot maintain a constant level of achievement.)

As well as stimulating the body, you also need to stimulate the mind. Talk to people, go to parties or throw your own, go out to the cinema, the theatre or to concerts. Become active in the community; write letters of complaint to the authorities, start a protest group or organize new projects for your local neighbourhood or charities. Try out new ideas and experiment and don't worry if they don't work out. This is your opportunity to find out what will work and what you will enjoy.

The extra energy available to you in the Virgin phase enables you to catch up on any work which fell behind during menstruation, as well as maintaining or often overtaking your normal workload. This is the time for you to look at new projects – any tasks left unfinished before menstruation need to be cleared away as soon as possible so that the fresh enthusiasm for new projects can be used to its best advantage.

During menstruation and the darkening phase, you may have lost sight of your priorities and direction in life so now is the time to analyse, organize and prioritize your life. It can be useful to write down the conclusions which you reach at this time, so that in the darker phases you can refer back to them. Look at your finances, home, relationships and goals and see if they can be managed in a better way.

This is a time when the intuitive ideas created at menstruation are given structure. The light of the Virgin is the light of wisdom, born from the depths of darkness to bring new life, awareness and structure into your life and to dispel fear and ignorance. Many women may feel unable to express the Virgin energies, constrained as they are by the social expectations of the 'correct' way for a woman to behave. The phase is dynamic and can in some ways be described as the 'masculine' aspect of the feminine, although this terminology may suggest that the two aspects are separate. Men can feel threatened by this phase, as it can encroach on their perceived 'territory' in society. The Virgin aspect of women is, however, as natural a part of being a woman as is being a mother.

As with all the phases, the Virgin phase needs to be balanced with the other aspects of the cycle. A woman who allows her Virgin aspect to dominate can become very career orientated and ambitious. She may repress her other aspects to become an 'honorary man', thereby enhancing her chances of getting to the top in her profession or in society. Such a woman may be very self-sufficient and self-contained and may find it difficult to give herself totally to a relationship or partnership. She may also be afraid of motherhood and unwilling, or unable, to allow herself to care for and nurture others. The intuitive, cyclic world of menstruation has little significance in her world.

Exercise: Virgin Meditation

Sit before a candle or a fire. Watch the light of the flame and feel its warmth. Allow the thoughts of the day to fade until you are aware only of the light. Close your eyes and hold the image of the flame before you. Feel the light in your body, travelling through your veins, and feel the exuberance of energy which travels with it. Feel the force of life within you, the pulse of light which is your life. Become aware that around you there are other flickers of light, the force of life within all things that live on the earth. When you feel ready, open your eyes and see the fire of your life reflected in the glowing light of the flame.

KEYWORDS

Dynamic / energy / intellect / brilliance / inspiration / fire / light / health / joy / body / exuberance / purity / unicorn / hound / lion / bull / huntress / warrior maid / Boudicca / Aphrodite / Athene / determined / analytical / self-confident / self-sufficient / strength / activity / sociability.

The Mother Phase

The Mother phase is a time of giving yourself and your love and abilities and of recognizing your link with the earth. In modern society, the mother may be viewed as a weak but necessary second-class citizen. Regardless of the advancements and achievements of women, the mother is seen as an instinctual animal, with her brain only able to cope with procreation and at the beck and call of bodily processes over which she has little control. Young women, and especially single mothers, are regarded as stupid for allowing themselves to become pregnant or as a drain on the finances of the state. The qualities of intelligence, strength and wisdom are no longer associated with motherhood in modern society and the abilities and virtues which they demonstrate in caring, selflessness and nurturing have been degraded to such a level that the women in this position no longer have respect or status. It is interesting to note that men who show these same abilities, attributes and tendencies are also victims of the same bias.

The Mother phase is a time of strength and energy, but unlike the Virgin, the energy is now expressed with a selfless quality, radiating rather than dynamic. The phase represents a pivot, balancing the outward expression of energy with the inner expression of love and caring. This phase can bring a feeling of contentment and wholeness built on a deep level of love and harmony. The Mother phase occurs around the time of ovulation and brings with it a sense of self-confidence and self-worth which enables you to offer support, encouragement, strength and help to others, with the confidence that you are able to both give and sustain it. The focus of the phase is outward, towards others and not towards yourself.

The Mother phase also brings with it a strong sex drive, which carries with it a deep love for the partner. Lovemaking brings joy in the giving of yourself totally to another and giving them pleasure. The care and love that you feel for your partner opens your awareness to a deeper level in which you yourself feel old beyond time and your partner becomes your child.

At this time community, actively caring and the desire to help other people can become important. The strength to achieve this is balanced by an inner, spiritual awareness of being part of the wonder of nature and the divine. Like the sexuality, the creative energies are also very strong and dreams may be very vivid with recurring images or themes.

INTERACTING WITH THE MOTHER ENERGIES

During the Mother phase, you may find that your clothes tend to express nature or earth mother themes in their style and colour. You may find that you want to express the energies in flowing ethnic clothes, using natural fibres and dyes, in floral patterns or

summer colours, or by using greens or reds to symbolize the life
energies flowing through you. Unlike the surface femininity of the
Virgin phase, the Mother phase holds a greater depth, so you may
find that your choice of clothes is less frivolous, more feminine and
more flowing. Allow your figure to show its curves but in a softer way
than in the Virgin phase. If you have a cleavage, show it! With your
deepening sexuality and inner confidence and strength, you may find
that you are paid more attention by men. You may want to wear more
jewellery in this phase and headier perfumes.

The best expression of the Mother phase is the body itself and you
may feel the need to be free of clothes altogether and only wear
jewellery. Obviously this is not recommended for work or for subzero
temperatures, but if you have the opportunity to walk naked around
your home or in the countryside, or even to just bare your breasts to
the sun and the breeze, use it as an expression of the openness of your
self to nature and the creative energies of life.

The Mother phase offers an opportunity for great joy in the giving of
yourself, your abilities, attention and help to other people. The Mother
holds the ability to take on responsibility for others, to care for and
love them and to offer them guidance, counselling and compassion.
Try to reach out to people and you may find that they will respond
to you more openly than they would at any other time of the month.
You may even find that people will approach you and tell you their
problems or ask for help and advice, without any prompting. Use your
strength and wisdom to offer help and advice, but do not force your
own views on others. One of the hardest things for mothers is to allow
their children to make their own mistakes. Reach out to friends and
family whom you have not seen for a while, write a letter or telephone.
Although it is often unnoticed in modern life, the mother is usually the
contact point for the whole family. It is the mother who remembers
birthdays, family traditions and anniversaries and who keeps the net
of the family strong by keeping in contact with those who have left
the original family home.

The Mother phase can be a time to visit your own mother, to see
her as the source of your own life as you may be the source of your
children's lives and to realize that although you are her child, you
are her equal as a woman and that you both share that bond which
goes beyond the differences in generation and outlook. With your
mother, you see the thread of life spiralling back into the past and
in you she sees that thread spiralling into the future. If you have
young children, try to do something a little special with them during
this phase; perhaps there are family or religious traditions which you
can teach them or perhaps you could arrange to spend a little more

time with them, helping them to learn. Children will often pick up the differences in your phases more quickly than adults.

The Mother phase carries a need for inner as well as outer expression. The phase can be very spiritual, bringing a feeling of harmony with life, nature and the divine. You may feel the need to be outside, to feel the forces of nature and life around you. If you have a garden or can find a quiet place amongst plants and trees, allow yourself time to sit quietly with nature and become part of it. Even if you live in a built-up area or a city, nature is still around you in the sky, the sun, the wind and rain, and the trees, plants, birds and insects which share our cities with us. You may well find that the awareness of nature is even more important for you if you do live in a city, rather than being surrounded constantly by the countryside. You may also find within yourself during this phase a deeper level of awareness and understanding of any animals with which you come into contact.

You may also wish to experience nature all around you at night time. If you have somewhere safe, experience the emotions and sensations which come with the darkness of night and the light of the stars or the moon.

The sexuality of this phase brings with it a strong creative drive. You may find that you suddenly want to make new things for the home, to redecorate or to create tidy order out of some chaos. If you have a garden, you can express these energies in nurturing and caring for your plants. Try to use your creative energies in producing something physical. This could be painting, design, craftwork, making music, writing or simply by cooking something a bit special. As you do this, be aware of the fact that you are creating something, even in a process which on the face of it may seem routine or mundane.

In this phase you may also find that you are more receptive to other people's ideas, often bringing new insights and a different perspective to them, and are also able to generate ideas of your own. These can be nurtured and brought into fruition during this time. If you find that some long term projects have started to drag, use the Mother phase to keep them going and to inject more impetus and enthusiasm into them.

The bright light of the Mother phase brings into the world creative energy from the dark womb of the Crone phase. Her light radiates outwards, encompassing all life. The bright moon is the dark moon made manifest, the whole of creation the manifest form of the divine. In the light of the full moon, renew your link with the divine in nature and within yourself. Ovulation at the time of the Full Moon brings a feeling of belonging to creation, of participating in creation and a joy of life. The Red Moon cycle with ovulation occurring with the dark moon sows the seed for the deep, inner knowledge and awareness to be brought out into the light of the manifest world.

A woman who represses the Mother energies can be unaware of the deep bonds of sharing and caring with other people. A woman who allows the energies to dominate her life can become passive, without ambition for her own life or without self-confidence in any matters beyond the home. She may often be exploited in a caring role, giving constantly of herself without regard for her own needs. She may hold onto family life as the total reason for her own existence and is often unable to adjust once her own children leave the family home.

Exercise: Mother Meditation

Sit in a garden or somewhere you can see a view of trees and plants. Notice the green colours, the shadows and the sunlight and gradually allow them to merge together. In your mind's eye, see a beautiful woman clad in a garment made from the landscape around you. Recognize yourself as part of her garment and feel her presence around you. Feel the peace and inner harmony which she brings and from deep within the love which bubbles up like a spring. All life around you is connected in the warp and weft of her garment and it shimmers in the creative energies which radiate from her. Become aware of those energies within yourself; feel your arms and hands pulse with the need and ability to love and care for all that you see. Allow those energies to spread beyond you, your sense of self no longer important when weighed against the need to comfort, protect and help soothe the pain and fears of others.

Bring your awareness gently back to your surroundings, retaining the feelings of love and peace.

KEYWORDS

Life / caring / compassion / love / nurturing / nourishing / strength / radiating / full moon / sustaining / giving / open womb / cow / bee / fertility / nature / earth / receptive / wisdom / counsel / fruit.

The Enchantress Phase

In some women, the Enchantress phase can be the most dramatic of all and can have the most impact on their daily lives. Like the Virgin phase, the Enchantress is a time of dynamic energy which gradually alters as the phase progresses; but unlike the Virgin energies, which are outward orientated, the Enchantress energies are directed inward. Physical strength and stamina gradually reduce and as the phase progresses you can become more agitated and restless, with an increasing need for activity but without real direction to this need. This restlessness can lead to anger, frustration, destructive self-analysis and guilt and self-reproach at the effect these symptoms may have on other people.

Although there is an increasing need to sleep, the mind is often too restless and hyperactive to relax. This mental activity reflects the increasing creative energy within the body, which may result in destructiveness unless it is allowed to find positive expression and form. Some women may find themselves less able to cope with the problems and pressures of life, especially as they near the end of the phase.

During the Enchantress phase, some women will find that their sexuality can become very intense. They can feel incredibly sensual but unlike the Virgin's sexuality which is funloving and outgoing, that of the Enchantress is at a more primal level. They can become self-assured in their sexual power, can tease or seduce and can be the original seductress whose power men find both tempting and frightening. The sexuality can become aggressive, demanding and even vampiric and is directed towards self-gratification. What can be a sensual energy at the beginning of the cycle can become eroticism towards the end. The Enchantress is more likely to participate in erotic practices, often with a sense of daring and a lack of responsibility.

During this time, women can become much more aware of their inner nature and may also feel the need to learn or practise something of a spiritual or intuitive kind. Energies generated during this phase can be tremendous, especially towards the end, and may be released as intense bursts of creation or destruction; by channelling and controlling the energy, however, it is possible to ensure that even the destructive forces can be turned to creative use. Psychic abilities may also increase at this time and dreams may take on magical themes and contain intense colours and emotions.

INTERACTING WITH THE ENCHANTRESS ENERGIES

During the Enchantress phase you may feel sensual, erotic and witchy, as though you could spin magic from your fingertips. Reflect these feelings in your appearance and clothes. You may wish to dress in dark colours using soft, flowing fabrics and black, sensual underwear to reflect your erotic nature. Use jewellery to reflect your magical feelings. Towards the end of the phase, you may find that your breasts and belly start to swell. As with the menstrual phase, dress in such a way as to draw the eye away from these features if you are uncomfortable about people seeing them, although with the increased sexuality and sensuality emerging in your body the larger breasts and belly can be welcomed as an expression of your womanhood.

With this phase comes an increasing need for awareness of the inner world, to interact with it and to learn more. You may find yourself more interested in esoteric, spiritual or psychological subjects, wanting to gain a greater understanding of them or you may wish to learn practical skills such as herbalism, aromatherapy, healing, astrology or dowsing. Search through bookshops and libraries to find a subject which satisfies the need you feel during this phase.

You may also find that you become more psychic or intuitive, experiencing predictive dreams and a need to find some type of structure or outlet for your feelings and experiences. There are many forms of divination such as Tarot cards, runes, tea leaves and scrying and it may be useful to try several of these methods until you find the one which best suits you. The Enchantress phase is a good time to learn about divination and the Hag phase is the best time to put your knowledge to use.

Towards the end of the Enchantress phase, awareness of the material world heightens; your senses may sharpen, setting off an avalanche of creative ideas and giving the world an almost surreal quality. You may feel more aware of the supernatural side to everything, gaining the impression of walking between two worlds, one visible and the other invisible.

During the Enchantress phase you may find yourself becoming increasingly restless, emotional and empathic, with reducing levels of concentration and thought processes which become increasingly illogical and emotional. If you find that you become hyperactive and agitated, try to learn relaxation or meditation techniques. The restlessness and frustration experienced during this phase can develop out of a restriction of the creative energies which build up. Relaxation may help you to cope on a daily basis, but ideally the energy needs to be redirected to a release in positive expression.

The Enchantress phase is a time of the withdrawal of physical energies and intellectual thought and the releasing of creative energies and intuitive thought. If these two aspects are not balanced, some women can experience dramatic mood swings. Repressed, the creative

energies find their own release, often in erratic bursts of physical and
emotional highs which can lead to demanding behaviour, insecurity
and unfocused hyperactivity. These highs can be followed by a swing
back to the withdrawn aspect of the phase, but this may be experienced
negatively as depression. This may result in erratic oscillation between
energy levels, with an inability to achieve consistency. By guiding the
creative energy and giving it an outlet in life, and by recognizing the
need for withdrawal, it is possible to smooth out the mood swings or
to see them in a more positive light.

If possible, try a simple creative pursuit at this phase in your cycle,
but be prepared to make a mess or to feel the need to destroy what you
have made. In this state, the final product is not important, but the
safe release of the energy is. The creative energies can appear in such
a rush that they lead to compulsive, almost manic behaviour to which
the release through a creative activity, and often the destruction of the
creation afterwards, can bring welcome relief. The energy build-up may
also be released through physical activity, but as the energy comes in
bursts, there is often no long term stamina. Methods of releasing, using
and guiding the often explosive creative energies of the menstrual cycle
will be considered in more detail in Chapter 5.

A woman in the Enchantress phase may be perceived as reproachful,
jealous, scolding and sharp-tongued. Her intolerance is often born out
of frustration and anger at the mundane world for not being able to
meet her needs. She wants to cut through the superfluous levels of
life and society in order to get to the true core. Such a woman will
frequently speak her own mind and tell the truth, often with little
regard for other people's feelings – although she may well later regret
having done so. Trivial, everyday annoyances which can be easily
dealt with during the other phases of the cycle can become blown up
out of all proportion, causing confusion and hurt to partners, family
and friends. She may become very penetrating and exactness becomes
very important to her, so that partners and family may feel that they
are unable to do anything right. The woman's manner at this time
reflects her underlying need for change and growth.

If you find from your Moon Dial that you experience this type of
behaviour on certain days during your cycle, try to avoid indepth or
heart-to-heart conversations on these days. You may find that you feel
less sociable and less willing to give people your time, expressing your
need to withdraw to your inner world. If possible, find time for yourself
to get away from people, to relax, to reconnect with the inner depths
of your being away from the torrent of your personality. Try using the
technique suggested for menstrual pain on page 82 to wash the tension
from your body or use the girdle visualization at the end of this chapter

to help to balance your energies. The Womb Awareness and Womb Tree exercises may also help you to reconnect your awareness with your body and its cycle, if you find yourself alienated from them.

Take time to look at your life and decide what changes need to be made. Use your intolerance to cut away the pressures and commitments and those aspects of relationships which are no longer necessary or which are the cause of problems. Decide to make a change in your life, however small, and look towards the Hag phase to pass from the old life into the new.

Towards menstruation, try to allow yourself more sleep and avoid jobs requiring concentration for long periods of time or those which demand fine co-ordination. You may also be living at a more emotional level, so try to organize your life so that the strains on your emotions are reduced.

As menstruation approaches, you may find that your sex drive becomes heightened. If you have a partner, try to make time to indulge in sex; the frustration and agitation felt at this time can manifest itself in an aggressive and demanding sexuality which can be unattractive for some men. The act of sex can release some of the frustration, but you may also find that you have a compulsive need for reassurance of your partner's love and fidelity. Rather than waiting for your partner to meet your needs, use your sexuality for romance, to seduce, to initiate, to become more adventurous and exciting. You may find that once unfettered and released, your wild sexuality may give you a level of experience which is normally submerged in everyday life.

The Enchantress phase also has a destructive aspect to its energies. If allowed to flow, a balance can be achieved, with these energies transformed into creation, allowed to flow harmlessly away or used to destroy in a controlled manner. These destructive energies can be used to clear away the old and unwanted from your life, breaking the ties which bind you to them. Some women may find that they tend to clean the house just before menstruation, subconsciously expressing the need to cut off the old cycle, clear away the debris and prepare for the new cycle. Often a change is necessary during this phase, whether in environment, routine or relationships, but it may well be change for its own sake. If the previous month has been traumatic for any reason, the need to cut off the old emotions may be expressed by changing your overall appearance. Having your hair cut or restyled, for example, can release the old you, allowing you to face the new month unencumbered by the past.

At other phases of the cycle change can appear frightening but in the Enchantress phase it is often necessary and welcomed. The phase holds a thread of truthfulness which allows you to look below the levels of illusion and realize how areas of your life can be changed. The Enchantress realizes that things are not static, that the death of the old is required before the birth of the new.

The Enchantress phase is a descent from the light, outward aspect of a woman's nature into the dark, inward aspect. If a woman is unable to make this descent, either by ignoring the change which she undergoes or by repressing the darker aspect of her nature, then the bond between her body, her mind and her cycle becomes broken. Energies which could be expressed by the conscious mind become trapped and forced to find their own expression in often self-destructive behaviour. Many women hate themselves at this time for the effect that their behaviour has on others and because their body is incapable of working and looking 'normal'. This process sets up a loop of destruction; the more a woman hates her true nature and her body, the more she denies expression to the phase's energies which then find outlets in behaviour which she hates in herself. To break the loop, a woman needs to find her own true nature and allow herself to act on it.

In the Enchantress phase, a woman's inner world becomes more important and closer to her conscious mind. Within her darkness lies the strong energies which can create or destroy. A woman who is unable to express the Enchantress energies can find that these energies take form in her life in a negative way. She may find herself with destructive tendencies which may occur mentally or physically, leading to self-inflicted injuries, violence, eating disorders or manic or compulsive behaviour. If, on the other hand, a woman allows the Enchantress energies to dominate her life, she may become agressive and domineering, with little thought or tolerance for other people. She may form shortlived relationships which have a purely sexual orientation, seeking constant change and variety. Such a woman may also be extremely creative, but in a compulsive, uncontrolled and unreliable manner.

Exercise: Enchantress Meditation

Sitting in a chair, relax and allow yourself to become aware of the darkness inside you. Within the darkness, you see a lens-shaped doorway from which streams brilliant white light into the darkness. As you watch, you notice that the stream of light emanating from the door is matched by a stream of darkness flowing into the door. At the doorway itself, the darkness becomes light and the light becomes darkness; creation and destruction are combined. You feel the interaction of the energies of dark and light within your mind and their constant movement. You feel the energy of your womb rise to your hands, pulsing in your fingertips. Accept within yourself the fact that the energy has the power to create or to destroy and that you have the control and responsibility for how it will be released. As you return to the outer world, acknowledge the darkness within yourself and the energy which stems from it.

KEYWORDS

Magic / witchy / psychic / intuitive / inner world / destruction / creation / Kali / Hecate / autumn / Persephone / serpent / dragon / owl / waning moon / descent / enchantress / seductress.

The Continuous Cycle

The need for a woman to feel connected with her true nature, her creative forces, her body and her place in nature can often express itself in negative behaviour if this need is ignored. By finding out what your needs are through the Moon Dial and then actively trying to meet them, you can learn to guide your energies and behaviour. There are of course some women who do need extra medical help and guidance for both mental and physical problems but a woman who becomes aware of her own problems and needs is more able to seek help of the most appropriate kind.

The individual energies or phases of the cycle should not be examined in isolation, but must be viewed as a whole. As with the moon's cycle, it is not possible to view the whole of the menstrual cycle at any one time; but some of the phases are visible and all the phases flow from one to another in a continuous movement. Any woman is her whole cycle; she is both its light and its darkness, but she can only be seen at any particular moment in terms of the phase she is in at the time. Women need to identify mentally with this cycle, to balance the different energies and phases and to use the best times of each month for the most appropriate tasks and lifestyle requirements.

As we have seen, there are optimum times during the month for certain activities. From your own Moon Dial records, you will be able to work out your own times of strengths and you will begin to realize that they are part of a repeating pattern. If you find that you cannot cope well with family or work at the time of menstruation, knowing that in a few days' time you will enter a phase of high mental and physical activity can relieve some of the mental pressure. For someone who uses creativity in their work, the change from a phase of active creativity to passivity can be frightening until they realize that the active phase will return or that the creativity has simply taken a different form. Most importantly, the Moon Dial emphasizes that there is nothing *wrong* with you.

The traditional, linear view of a period of time – say a year – could be described as a series of jobs or projects, each of which will be carried through with times of high input and low input until they are completed. If you view the year as a sequence of repeating cycles, however, it should be possible to arrange the tasks so that each receives the most appropriate attention and energy at each phase in your cycle; thus work can be maintained at high levels of achievement and ability throughout the year. The Maiden phase may be used for analysis, developing new projects and raising enthusiasm; the Mother phase is the time to maintain projects and support relationships; the Enchantress phase is used for learning and high creativity; and finally the Hag phase for removing the old and outdated and developing new insights and ideas. Although this approach is clearly not always possible when working to rigid deadlines or in pressurized circumstances, for less rigid work or longer term projects the active use of your cycle can produce your most inspired ideas and work and give you the most satisfaction.

The four phases of your cycle also provide you with an opportunity to assess your life once a month and to make changes where necessary. The Enchantress phase is the time to analyse your life in detail and decide what needs to be changed; the Hag phase is the time to grieve for the old life and to mentally accept the change; the Virgin phase is the time to make the change physically within your life; and the Mother phase allows your change to come to fruition.

By being true to all sides of your nature, you acknowledge that you can be self-confident, active and strong, that you can nurture without being weak, that you can be wild and instinctual or calm and reasoning and that you have a darkness within, a depth beyond the mundane world.

Exercise

After reading this section and forming your Moon Dials, you may find it useful to re-read the story of *The Awakening* as a summary of the energies of the menstrual cycle.

EXPANSION OF THE MOON DIAL

The Moon Dial can become more than just a series of observations, but rather a source of expression of your monthly cycle, even a piece of living art. At the end of the section entitled 'The Moon Dial' it was suggested that colour should be used with the Moon Dial to enhance the different phases. This idea can be taken a stage further to produce a symbolic wheel of your own energies.

Using your coloured Moon Dial as a basis, including the moon phases but without the numbering, the wheel becomes a symbol of your cycle rather than a vehicle for observation. Add to the Moon Dial any symbols, colours and images which express how you feel about each phase. Use phrases or words, photographs or natural objects if you feel unable to draw. You may like to refer to the keywords listed above after each section on the different phases or study Figure 8. Your symbol can be as simple or as complicated as you wish; it can be drawn on paper, on wood or on stone and made to any size. Complete the image with a small central circle representing your inner self. The image created represents your own cyclic energies and by using it in meditation or simply by looking at it, you can remind yourself of all of your aspects.

You may also express your Moon Dial symbol in a three-dimensional form, perhaps a girdle or necklace. Choose different beads to represent each of the moon's phases and tie them, equally spaced, onto a leather thong. Use different coloured threads, beads and artefacts to represent the different energies and associations which you have developed with each phase and tie them onto the thong between the moon phase beads. You may find it easier to adapt an existing belt or necklace. If you can, try to make each section of the girdle/necklace during the appropriate phase of your cycle – this will make it easier to express your feelings about the phase, rather than simply trying to remember. Tying the two ends around your hips or around your neck completes

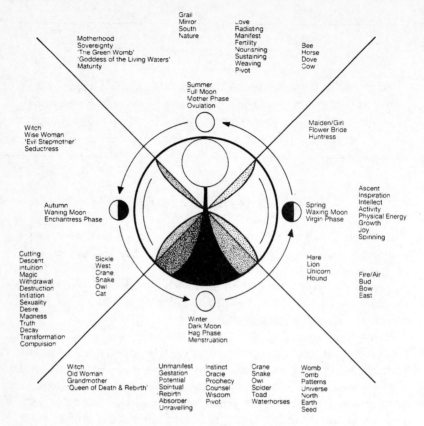

Figure 8   Moon Dial associations

the circle of your cycle and standing within the loop, you are at the point of balance of the cycle's energies.

Exercise: Girdle Visualization

Sit wearing your girdle and allow yourself to slowly relax. Become aware of the inner darkness and feel comfortable and poised. Visualize yourself standing in the centre of a huge dark plain. Above you, you notice the tiny pinpricks of stars in the dome of the sky. In front of you, in the east, the sky brightens with the light of a rising crescent moon. Allow images which you associate with this phase of your cycle to appear in front of you; they may include animals, colours, music, people, goddesses or scenes. Allow them all to appear on the plain, perhaps some in daylight, others in moonlight. Feel the energies associated with this phase rise through your body. You may find that you wish to interact in some way with the images.

When you feel ready, return to your original position and turn to the south. As you turn, feel the energies in your body flow and alter. Before you, you see a large harvest moon in an ultramarine sky. Allow images associated with this phase to appear on the plain and the energies to rise in your body. When ready, turn to the west and do the same as you watch the setting horns of the waning moon. Finally, face the darkness of the north with its stars and allow your awareness to give shape and form to the energies and feelings there. Be aware of the light phases of the moon behind you and to your sides and then turn your awareness towards yourself at the centre of the plain.

Around you are your energies and personalities through the month. Recognize yourself as Virgin, Mother, Enchantress and Hag and realize that these selves are all equally part of your self. As you stand at the centre, be aware that you stand outside these personalities that although the waves of energies ebb and flow around you, the essence which is you stands solidly at the centre. Push your awareness back out into the cycle and feel the energies around you, realizing that you no longer need to be like a boat buffeted by the currents and waves turning you every which way, but that you are now able to read the currents, to set your sail and rudder and use harmony with the energies to steer your own course.

See encircling the edge of the plain a huge, multicoloured snake which ripples with the flow of energies. Become aware of the girdle encircling your hips and allow it to overlap with the scene around you as a symbol of the cycle of energies which you hold in balance. When ready, slowly bring your awareness back to your body.

In this way the girdle becomes an active link with your cycle and a way for you to balance or reconnect with the energies of your cycle.

The expression of your cycle will change throughout your life and so at some time another symbol will need to be painted or the girdle or necklace reworked. These objects are not intended to be static; they are not intended to pin down your cycle, but are rather a way of expressing your cycle at that time. At the end of menstruation, whether through menopause or pregnancy, the expression needs to be unmade and a new one found. The object itself is not sacred, but the cycle it expresses and the process of making it are. The last threads or beads of a grandmother's girdle could be woven into her daughter's girdle and the mother could make her daughter's first girdle starting with some threads of her own. The girdle then becomes not only a symbol of the cyclic nature of women but also a living tradition.

FURTHER WORK

After completing the exercises in *Red Moon*, you may wish to continue working on and with your menstrual energies. This book can only scratch the surface of the ideas and inspirations linked to the menstrual cycle and there is much for women to find out individually, or to relearn as a group. The concept of the journal can be taken beyond a few months and used to reflect longer term influences on your cycle.

During the course of a year, see if the season has an effect on your phases. Notice if the moon going through different zodiac signs has an influence on your cycle and energies. If you are with a group of women on a long term basis or have a close relationship with a woman, see if your cycles resonate. If you become a mother, note if the energies of your cycle have changed. Also note if your cycle changes orientation depending on your aspirations and goals in life.

The longest term influences on a woman's cycle are clearly the phases of her own life. Identification of the menstrual phases and energies will enable her to pass through each of her life phases with more ease. The change from Maiden to Mother to Crone will become easier to accept in the knowledge of the turning of the cycle, the living to the full of the energies of the phase she has just left and the anticipation of the energies to come in the new phase. By experiencing the whole cycle within herself, a woman is able to see the cycle and empathize with it in the girls, mothers and old women she sees around her and to perceive that cycle as a continuity through time.

FIVE

The Creative Moon

WOMEN'S CREATIVITY

The concept of the moon as a source of the creative spirit was one of the earliest ideas expressed by humankind and can still be found surviving in some cultures today, as well as echoed in legend and mythology. The link between women's creativity and the moon was observed in the repeating cycle of creative energy which changed shape and form throughout a woman's menstrual cycle. These energies gave each woman the capacity to create, that is, to bring into being the unmanifest, whether an idea, understanding or life itself. The creative energy formed a bridge between the tangible world and the intangible and found expression through the intellect, the emotions, the intuition, the subconscious and the body, depending on the particular phase of the woman's cycle. Women's creativity, sexuality and spirituality were seen to arise from their bodies and its rhythms, and the creative energies connected to their sexuality were recognized as underlying the menstrual cycle which renewed life itself each month.

Many modern women consider themselves completely uncreative and may actively turn away from anything which they consider as 'creative'. The creative energies, however, are not just confined to painting pictures, playing an instrument or writing poetry, but are active throughout a woman's life, regardless of whether or not their expression is viewed as creative. All women have the capacity to create, but how they relate to this potential depends on their own awareness of their creative energies and the links with their bodies, sexuality and spirituality. Many women have a limited view of creativity, not because of their perception of their own abilities or inabilities but because of the restricting view which society places the *products* of creativity. Creativity is not expressed in the product but rather in the *process* of giving form. It is the giving of form to the experience of your inner self in relation to the world around you, whether in a tangible form such as the production of a child or a painting or in an intangible form such as an idea, a relationship or a dance.

The changing shape of her sexuality through the month changes a woman's perception of life, altering her awareness and experiences and her expression of the creative energies within her. The energies of the Virgin phase are initiating and visionary, those of the Mother phase physical and emotional, the Enchantress phase dynamic and intuitive and the Hag phase instinctive and spiritual. These energies arise through the woman's body and mind each month, offering no distinction between the creative energies and her sexuality and sensuality. At the height of each woman's sexual and erotic experiences in her monthly cycle, her perception of the world can produce the most creative and spiritual expressions.

The cycles of sexuality, spirituality and creative awareness become inseparable in a woman who lives her true nature. This nature is to *express* her awareness, to create form for her needs and feelings, to celebrate her joy of life and enjoyment of her body and to express the relationship between herself and the worlds in which she walks. If women's creativity is seen as a process of reflecting the experience of life and the true nature of a woman, this perspective does not restrict the view of 'art', as a product of creativity, to a few abstract paintings in an expensive gallery but rather widens it to include all aspects of a woman's life and capabilities.

'Art' may be any way in which a woman's creative energies are expressed, with all forms of expression having equal validity regardless of their physical form or the relative ability of the woman to express it. An amateur painting with little technical skill is as valid as a professional painting of great skill, and the writing of a love poem is as valid as creating a solution to a problem or baking a cake. If 'art' is seen as the expression of the creative energies through the physical and inner experience and awareness of life, then the division between art and life dissolves and all aspects of life become art. In museums, the modern person is often struck by the beauty of the decoration with which ancient cultures covered the most basic and menial artefacts. For these earlier cultures, art was an expression of life and was reflected in their own lives at every level.

In modern society, the expression of the creative energies has become restricted by the perception of the created product. Often, the product is required to have 'meaning', an intellectual rationale, in order to have perceived value, and the experience of both producer and receiver add negligible value to the worth of the art form. This restriction of the perceived value of art has led to a society in which many of the traditional women's creative forms have lost respect and worth. The modern view of art is one of technical skill and intellectual perception beyond the capabilities of the ordinary person. The traditional women's arts are, however, widespread and are available to all.

Traditional Women's Arts

The traditional women's creative skills were originally an expression of the creative energies applied to the areas of survival, tradition, beauty, understanding, motherhood, insight and wisdom, and reflected the women's experience and interaction with life. In the past, these skills and the creative capacity of women were respected and considered vital for the survival of the people and were recognized as a reflection of the divine. Women provided the stability and the source of the community; women created the home as a place of security, safety, comfort and belonging and in many cultures, especially nomadic ones, the woman would actually build the home, providing shelter for her family and man.

Women also provided food by gathering or growing crops and cultivating the land. They cooked, thereby creating food from sources which would have been inedible without this treatment, and preserved and stored food to enable survival through the winters. Through their knowledge of plants, women were able to create healing and well-being. Women used the resources around them to make the things necessary for survival and comfort; skins were made into housing, clothing and decoration and later the fleeces of domesticated sheep and goats were spun into wool and woven into fabric.

It was often women who traditionally made the pots for storage, cooking and carrying water and the mats and baskets woven from reeds and branches. All aspects of their work and skills were decorated to reflect the beauty of the world around them and often these tasks would take on a devotional role in the religious expression of the women. These decorative skills were not important to the direct survival and physical well-being of the family, but they brought the awareness of beauty into the community and later became important features in trade between the different settlements.

Women also created the family; not only through the birth of children who would continue the race but also through the concept of belonging. The relationships founded by the women became a source of structure, providing help, support and caring in time of need. Women's ability to create the continuance of life brought about the concepts of continuity and of ancestry, and women were also responsible for passing on the skills and traditions necessary for survival to their children. The woman helped create understanding in the child of the role of humanity within nature, creating the future traditions and personality of the community.

Even with the increase in male dominance, the creative abilities of women were still sought after, although they largely lost their original respect and place in society. The woman became a producer of products, of the home, of heirs, of clothing and food and anything which she produced immediately became the property of a male. Her 'magical' ability to create was overshadowed by the ownership of what she created. The active expression of a woman's creative energies through her intellect or spirituality in society, however, became closed to her. Women still retained importance in the production of children and in particular, male heirs, but their ability to help create the personality and understanding of their children was taken over by male society.

Until the 1960s, women as creators of the home and of children still had value in western society, although their intellectual, sexual, spiritual and creative expressions were restricted, often reduced to the idea of 'keeping their husbands and families happy'. Women still used their skills to provide food, to make clothing and artefacts and to create a family and home but the importance of these functions, except in times of war, was seen as very much secondary to the work and role of the male.

After the 1960s and the rise of feminism, the role of women in society underwent a discernible change. Women began to demand the opportunity to use their abilities in areas other than the home. The image of the intellectual woman with her creative abilities applied to communication, problem solving or the forming of ideas, structures and organization began to achieve some recognition. To gain this recognition, however, women had to compete with men on their terms and the result of this battle was the degeneration of the last matriarchal expression of motherhood and homemaker. The traditional creative skills of women became viewed by women themselves in male terms, as being of less importance than 'proper' work and even demeaning. Women who did not wish to give up the traditional motherhood role came under increasing pressure from both sides; by men for not pulling their weight in the financial world and by the 'new' women for letting the side down. In the 'freedom' of feminism, the role of women became polarized by society into the 'good' or 'bad' mother and the 'good' or 'bad' working woman.

The image of motherhood as the source and strength of society has become lost and at worst mothers are now viewed as a financial drain. Hospital orientated maternity care and childbirth reduce a woman's control over her body and can make the experience of childbirth no more than a cost-effective production line. Society's image of the mother is no longer one of strength but of a soft woman, lacking any personal or intellectual fortitude. Thus women who leave jobs in order to have a family often have great difficulty in finding new work when they wish to return to the job market. Although companies must legally offer equal opportunities, there is still a lingering feeling that to train a woman, who will want to leave her career in order to raise a family at some time in the future, is to waste money. The images of women's other traditional creative skills have also declined in status. Where they were once the means of survival, the expression of the experience and understanding of life, they are now reduced in stature to hobbies with little worth to modern society.

The creative energies and abilities of women have much to offer society and modern women are beginning to have the opportunity to express them once again in areas to which women in the past had access, as well as in areas previously beyond the experience of women. There are, however, no strict roles for a woman and the expression of her creative energies. Her use of her energies through motherhood, as a company director or as a wise woman are all valid and all a part of the nature of woman. For society in general to accept all the expressions of a woman's energies, whether Maiden, Mother, Enchantress or Hag, women need firstly to recognize these aspects within themselves and secondly to permit and accept them within other women.

AWAKENING THE CREATIVE ENERGIES

The creative energies arise in the menstrual woman through her body, her sexuality and sensuality and through her awareness. The word 'sensuality' is used here to denote the awareness of the world through the senses and the body. The link between a woman's body and her mind means that the creative energies may be woken by the mind, through visualization or thought, or by the body, through its interaction with the world around it; it means that some methods of awakening the creative energies may also be used to release those energies.

Awakening the creative energies through the body depends on a woman's awareness of her body and her understanding and acceptance of it. Through the use of the Moon Dials, you can recognize patterns in your sexual/creative energy, the way you react to it and the ways in which you express it either consciously or subconsciously. Understanding that certain behaviour at certain times in your cycle can be an expression of your creative energies is the first stage towards actively awakening and using the energies in everyday life.

Some women may already be consciously aware of the creative 'urge' in their lives and the Moon Dials offer them a guide to their monthly pattern. Women who are not aware of this urge still experience the changing patterns of the creative energies through their menstrual cycles, but may be unaware that what they are experiencing is the flow of these energies and that they are in fact actively being creative in their lives. In Chapter 4, some of the possible expressions of the creative energies in the four phases of the menstrual cycle were considered and the following sections will examine in more detail specific ways in which the energies can be deliberately released.

Before being able to release the creative energies, a woman must first be able to awaken those energies or to recognize their existence when they arise in the month. During the month the creative energies change quality and orientation; the outwardly radiating energy of the Mother phase is different in its expression from that of the inward depth of the Hag phase. A woman who is aware of these changes realizes that she does not lose her creativity at certain times, but rather that it changes its expression. By recognizing this, a woman may accordingly adjust the way in which she lives her life, enabling her to get the best from her monthly cycle. The creativity of women lies within the *flow* of their sexual and creative energies and to restrict the flow is to restrict the expression of the creative nature.

The simplest way in which a woman may awaken her creative energies is to become more sensual and more aware of her body and its interaction with the world around it. This may be achieved by making yourself notice the sensations of your body and the way it reacts to textures and tastes, smells and temperature. Notice details like the feel of your clothing on your skin, the sensation of sunlight on your body. Experience the world around you through your skin; walk barefoot or naked if you can. Heighten your awareness of sounds and scents, take pleasure in the sights, shapes and colours of the world around you and feel alive! If you have a partner or family, be aware of their touch and their smell. Allow your mind to become aware of your womb, feeling its position in your body. You may notice that during the month this heightened sense of awareness will arise of its own accord, accompanying a period of creativity.

Use movement to music or rhythm to heighten your awareness of your body and its ability to express your inner emotions. If you are uncomfortable with dancing, choose a familiar piece of music with a steady rhythm and *allow* your body to respond. Set aside the embarrassment and mental restrictions which you keep in place in everyday life and give your body the freedom to move without restraint. As you respond to the music, use your voice, perhaps with cries and calls, to further express the feelings which the music awakens. Your movement does not need to be complicated and often the body will find the movement which suits it. Even a simple shift in body weight from one foot to the other can heighten the awareness of the body. As you dance, feel sexual, alive and receptive to the energies in your body.

The female link between sexuality and creativity means that the act of making love to a partner arouses and awakens the creative/sexual energies in a woman. If you are sexually active, notice the heightened sensuality which you experience during lovemaking and the effects which sex has on your feelings, moods and everyday life.

The heightened sense of awareness may also be experienced in your interaction with the natural world. Be aware of the sense of life around you and the sensations and emotions which it evokes within you. Touch and be touched by the life around you. Experience nature at night and notice the change in your perceptions which the darkness, the stars and the moon bring.

All these methods of awakening the creative energies can be used separately or in various combinations in the course of everyday life. To combine all these methods – the heightened sense of awareness experienced in nature, dancing to rhythmic music and the act of making love – is to form the basis of the ancient fertility rites.

The creative energies may also be awoken through the mind as well as the body. The experiences of life can trigger them and often a dramatic event, like a death in the family, can produce bursts of creativity which are compulsive in their need for release. Become more aware of your mental as well as physical interaction with the environment. Sometimes an event, a shape, a sight or a sound will spark a rush of creative energy, taking its own form in your mind as an idea, a picture, an insight or a piece of music. Try to discover how other people express their creative energies; visit art galleries and sculpture, craft fairs, opera, theatre, concerts, traditional folk events, architectural sites and ancient earthworks and notice how people express their own creativity in the everyday world, in cooking, gardening, caring and loving. You may find that their creative expression awakens a corresponding need within you and brings the inspiration to focus that creativity. View all expressions of other people's creativity with an open mind and release any preconceptions of what you think art should be.

Visualization can be a strong tool in this process. The 'Awareness of your Womb' visualization on page 78 draws the mind's attention to the womb and then allows the energy up into the hands ready for release or expression. The visualization is simple and with practice can be used at any time when the need to reconnect with the creative energies arises. Sometimes the simple visualization of an image or a symbol which represents the creative energies enables a woman to identify with it and to feel it within her. The Womb Tree is an example of an image which may be used for this purpose. As you find out more about the symbols of your own menstrual cycle, you may find images which will allow you to establish a link between your mind and your creative energies.

The 'Awareness of your Womb' exercise used visualization to promote creative expression in the physical world. The visualization which follows uses the interaction between the mind and the image of the Womb Tree to enhance creative mental expression in ideas, insight, inspiration and understanding. The spark of life of the idea children is conceived in the womb of the mind; some will be given a physical form whilst others become part of the growth and development of the mother.

Both the 'Awareness of your Womb' visualization and the following one may be used at any time during the month, but you may find that you are drawn to one or the other during particular phases.

Exercise

The following visualization allows you to open your mind to accept the flow of creative energies in the form of ideas. You may find that you will receive these ideas during the visualization or afterwards in everyday life. These are your idea children; they may be allowed to grow and may eventually be given form in the manifest world or they may be absorbed back into yourself.

Sit comfortably and allow yourself to relax. Be aware of your womb and feel it lying in the darkness of your body. Draw your attention into the darkness and gradually become aware of standing in front of your Womb Tree. Take time to notice the details of the tree and the current phase of the moon in its branches.

Before you lies the pool of water and, standing on tiptoe, you reach up to touch a branch which stretches out across it. As you touch the branch, the leaves rustle and you hear your name whispered in their movement. Looking into the leaves you see a small white dove with a pale pink breast looking out at you with deep orange eyes. In a single graceful movement, it launches itself from the branch and glides across the pool to land at the base of the Womb Tree. The image of the white dove standing at the base of the moonlit tree causes hints of memory to stir in the depths of your mind.

A soft female voice inside your head welcomes you and invites you to cross the waters of life and enter the darkness of birth. As the voice speaks, you become aware of a star of light on your forehead, shining brightly. Across the pool, a sphere of white light grows around the dove, washing its feathers in flames of light. The dove rises to hover in front of the tree trunk.

Tentatively, you touch the water with your foot, expecting to sink, but instead you find that you are able to walk across it. When you reach the tree you find that an entrance has opened in the trunk and you follow the dove into its depths. You stand in the dark, feeling the walls of the womb surrounding you with its pulsing energy. You stretch your arms upwards, allowing the flow of light and love to pour from the dove through your body. You become aware of your belly and breasts, swollen as though in pregnancy. You feel poised and balanced, sensing the seeds of inspiration, as yet unformed, resting inside you.

Remain in this position until you feel ready to return. Allow the presence of the dove's light and the Womb Tree to gradually fade and your body to return to its normal size. Become aware of your body sitting and breathe deeply as you open your eyes. You may still feel the residual light from the dove resting within you.

Very often in the modern world, time spent being creative is given a low priority in people's lives. By recognizing that your nature is creative and is linked to your mind through your body and its cycles, you are able to become aware of your creative potential. Unless you spend time connecting with and responding to your creative energies, however, they remain simply potential. Restriction of the creative energies in general can cause a sense of isolation, staleness, low inspiration, lack of sexuality and impaired awareness of the physical world. Repression of the creative energies at times when they are dynamic can lead to irritability, frustration, destructive tendencies and compulsive behaviour. It is therefore important for each woman to find time in her life to become aware of her own creative abilities and expressions if she is to be true to her nature.

RELEASING THE CREATIVE ENERGIES

The creative energies need to be released constructively if harmony and balance are to be achieved and the following sections consider a number of different ways in which the energies may be expressed. These sections are not intended to be comprehensive, but offer suggestions and ideas which may be tried and accepted, rejected or built upon. By expressing her creative energies, a woman accepts, becomes more aware of and celebrates these energies of womanhood. The more a woman allows her energies to flow, the more readily they become available to her and the more obvious become the methods of release appropriate for that particular woman.

Any product resulting from the process of release, the mode of expression or performance is secondary in importance to the release itself. Any action or experience in life can be an expression of the creative energies, if you are aware that you are interacting with your creative ability. Some expressions of the energies will feel natural or easy to do whilst others will require perseverance and practice and it is important to find methods of expression which suit you. By learning those expressions which give you most satisfaction and those which come most easily at the time when you are feeling at your most creative, you may manage your cycle and your life to make the most of your creative abilities. You then learn to live within your cycle rather than beyond it.

Enthusiasm and creativity are closely linked and there may be a compulsion to release the creative energies when inspiration sparks an idea or when the need to create arises. As a phase of dynamic creativity passes, the enthusiasm for an idea will often also pass unless the idea is acted upon. Although the idea or act of expression could be developed at a later date, it becomes more difficult to awaken the same enthusiasm which came at the origin. Knowing when your phases of creativity arise in your cycle enables you to prepare or organize time so that you are able to express the energy when it does arise and ensures that you do not lose enthusiasm or feel frustrated or blocked. Between highly dynamic phases of creativity, the expressions of the other phases may be used to build upon that produced in the dynamic times.

The products which arise from the first expressions may not live up to expectations but technical skill develops with practice and from each individual expression you learn something more about your energies and abilities. The product of the raw, experimental stage often holds more power and beauty than the later expressions which are refined by the restrictions of conscious skills and rules.

Exercise

Look through your Moon Dials and note the ways in which you already express your creative energies, whether consciously or subconsciously. Note if you have times when you particularly want to paint, to write, play music, make love, dance, cook, clean, garden, be with nature or care for others. Notice how you cope with your creative urges; do you act on them? What are your needs? Do you restrict your expression and do you have times of frustration? You will find that the days of highest sexuality and creativity tend to coincide in your cycle and that these days are very active and dynamic. You may also find times when your creativity is less physical and is expressed internally.

The information from your Moon Dials can be used as a basis for experiment. If you find that you are expressing your energies in one form, try another outlet, possibly one suggested in the sections below. If you are not sure about which form of expression would suit you, try several different methods during your different phases and note their effect on you. By experimenting, you will expand your view of your own creative ability and will redefine what you see as a creative expression.

If you have a regular dynamic creative time or phase, try to allocate some time to actively express it. It may be useful to keep materials, equipment, music, etc. ready so that you can avoid the frustration of having to indulge in lengthy preparation or finding that you do not have the correct materials. Try not to force your creativity; it will flow readily when its orientation during the phase is recognized, accepted and used. There will be times in the month when you feel that the energy has disappeared. It may be that the orientation of the energy is different from that expected, the method of expression no longer suits you or that other influences such as relationships, stress or health are burying the link between your mind and your true nature.

Most importantly, *try something*. Give the energy the chance to be released. If you have an idea or sudden insight, write it, paint it, give it a form in some way and you may find that it starts an avalanche of inspiration. If you want to dance, give in to the urge and dance! The gift of womanhood is to give birth to knowledge, understanding and insight in the material world in whatever form a woman chooses. Have confidence in your ability as a woman to create.

The following sections are divided into ways of expression through the hands, the body, the mind and the environment. The division of these expressions into the four categories is merely to provide a point of reference, as often each expression is a mixture of all of them.

Expression through the Hands

TRADITIONAL SKILLS

The simplest way of expressing the creative energies is through your hands and many of the traditional women's skills use this form. Women have for generations spun, sewn, woven, knitted, embroidered, made tapestries, baked, cooked, constructed baskets, rugs, clothes and pots and decorated the everyday objects of their lives. These crafts may now tend to be treated as old-fashioned or frivolous, but they offer a woman a fairly simple and traditional means of creating and making beauty. The products of these crafts enhance the world of the woman herself and of those around her; she creates form, beauty, sustenance and comfort from the simple raw materials. The baked cake, the child's booties, the tapestry footstool and the embroidered napkin are all expressions of the woman's creative energies and her desire and need to allow them to flow. Awareness of this often makes the recipient of a handmade gift more appreciative and respectful of the object which they have been given.

ART

The more recognized and socially appreciated expressions of the creative energies released through the hands are, for example, the skills of painting, drawing, sculpting, woodworking and crafting ceramics and jewellery. Many people are reluctant to attempt these art forms, as they are perceived as in some way 'special' and beyond an ordinary person's ability.

Art is one of the oldest forms of human record; it expresses the artist's view of themselves and their interaction with the world around them. The inspiration for art comes from the awareness of life and the outside world and it is the inner world which takes these experiences and forms them into a new creation. Everyday tools and utensils can become objects of beauty, decorated with lines, spirals, flowers and animals or inlaid with precious stones and metals. To ancient cultures whose art reflected their spiritual awareness, the modern environment would seem dull and lifeless.

Use art to express your own feelings at your time of creativity. There is no need to start with a particular idea of what you are going to paint or make; just express yourself through the colours, textures and form. You may find, though, that with the phase of creative energies comes a mental image of a final product, which may be in a medium totally different from the one you are used to, in which case you should experiment with the new medium.

Art can physically express the inner needs and imbalances of a person and can be used as a method of healing. Often the most creative and intuitive works of art have been created by people who have mentally withdrawn from the everyday world. The source of the creative energies lies beyond the conscious reactions to life and will often emerge at times of withdrawal, whether through menstruation, illness or trauma, to give healing to the personality. This introspection can be seen as a pause in a woman's life, the opportunity to be still and to allow the creative energies to heal by giving shape and form to her inner needs. By giving them form, the problems can be acknowledged, transformed or released, leading to healing and strength. The product of this expression may be kept as a representative of the result of healing through creation or it may be destroyed as a symbol of the ending of the old life and a celebration of the new.

HEALING

The expression of the creative energies through the hands for the purpose of healing may also be found in the concept of the laying on of hands. This concept comes very naturally to women, as they have a greater tendency to express their caring, love and affection for people through touch. You may find that during the month you become aware that your hands tingle or feel warm. This energy can be expressed or released in the creation of healing and well-being as easily as through painting, cooking or knitting.

Try experimenting with this at a time when you feel that the healing energies are easy to raise. Find a comfortable position to sit in and become aware of your own sexuality and creative energy. You may want to use an image or a symbol which you connect with the current phase of the month to help to raise your awareness of the energies, or you may wish to perform the 'Awareness of your Womb' visualization. Allow the energy to slowly build in your hands, making them feel warm and radiating heat. Hold your hands in front of you, palms facing each other but not touching, and experiment with trying to make them feel hotter or cooler. Gradually pull your hands apart until you can no longer feel the heat and then bring them back together. If you are not going to release the energy in healing, place your hands on the ground or under running water and allow the energy to dissipate.

If you do want to release the energy in healing, hold your hands just above the area which needs care so that the person you are helping can feel the warmth of your hands. Concentrate on the energy within your hands and as you breathe out feel the energy flow into that person, directing it with feelings of love and caring. You may wish to use a prayer or a spiritual image to help you in the process.

The energy can be released in a more general way to give an enhanced sense of well-being. This can be done in any form which feels suitable; for instance, by holding a person's hand, giving them a hug or through massage.

To become a healer in any professional sense, a woman will clearly need far more guidance and training than can be offered briefly in this book. This does not mean that a woman should not practise using her energies to help and care for the well-being of her partner, family, friends and pets. To offer a general healing to your family is to offer them your love.

Expression through the Body

BODY ART

A woman experiences the world through her body and her sensuality and is also able to express that experience using her body. For women, art is not just a product outside themselves but is communicated through the body itself. This connection between the mind, the body and the surroundings means that the body and the space around it become an expression of the woman's awareness. This expression can be evident in clothes, hairstyles, adornment, body painting, music, sex, performance or the decoration of the home, the work place or the landscape.

The decoration of the naked body with paint and natural objects is one way for a woman to express her feelings of interconnectedness with nature. Nakedness allows a woman to reach the heights of her awareness of her body and of her sensuality and through that sensuality she becomes part of her surroundings. A naked woman is not truly naked, but rather clothed in the living earth around her. The rise of Christianity altered the concept of a woman's sensuality from an expression of interaction with the divine into one of temptation and evil. The female body became the object of men's desires and fears and it can be difficult in modern society to break away from these associations.

To express the creative energies publicly through the decoration of nakedness is not acceptable in modern society, so women can only express their feelings, moods and sexuality in the ways in which they cover their nakedness. In Chapter 4, the section on 'The Moon Dial and Everyday Life' suggested a number of ways in which a woman could identify with her monthly phases through the way she dresses. By seeking conscious expression for her inner awareness in clothes, a woman becomes freed from the restraints of fashion and the expectations of men.

DANCE

The concept of the body as an expression of the link between the outer and inner worlds may also be found in dance. Dance has a long history of use in religious rites and ceremonies and through dance a participant was able to forge a link with the inner world and the divine and to invoke the energies and mysteries beyond everyday survival. For women, dance was a natural expression of their cyclic duality.

The oldest dances tend to be circular dances with simple rhythms and actions to be repeated. Echoes of these ancient circle dances can be found in folk stories of dancers being turned into stone, forming stone circles, in the 'faery rings' supposedly formed by the actions of dancing faeries and in the traditional treading of mazes at seasonal festivals. Dancing women used the expression of the body to link them to the cycles of the seasons and the moon and to the spirit world. The dancing would often climax in a state of trance or exhausted ecstasy in which the restraints of the intellect were released.

The treading of the maze was a slightly more complicated form of the circle dance, in which a line of dancers would make their way along a spiral path to the centre of a designated pattern and then dance their way outwards, unravelling the spiral once again. These dances reflected the journey of the moon into darkness and its re-emergence into light, the spiralling of life in towards death

and its return to new life, the path of the seasons as the life force
and light withdrew from the land and returned in the spring, and the
path of the mind in the menstrual cycle which turned inwards to the
darkness of the subconscious and inner world before returning to the
outer world.

To dance the maze in the spring, at the full moon or at the birth
of a child was to express the part of humanity in the rhythm of the
universe and the source of life. To dance at the dark of the moon,
at autumn time or following a death was to return to the dark mother
in order to bring her wisdom and insight into the manifest world. The
dancers became a symbol of the divine feminine and were themselves
part of that symbol. The symbol of the dance remained the same but
the interpretation of the symbol changed, depending on when and
why it was danced.

Even in the modern world, it is easy to lose oneself to the rhythm
of a dance, whether it is in a disco or formal dance or at home listening
to your own music. In dance, the mind responds at a deeper, more
instinctual level, enabling everyday thoughts to be lost in the rhythm
of the music. As the dance takes over, the intellectual restrictions and
inhibitions of the conscious mind dissolve, allowing expression to the
inner self through the body and the creative energies. A dancer trusts
her body to the rhythm; any attempt to concentrate on the beat or
the dance movements may result in the loss of the rhythm. Dance
becomes the art of the body, the expression of the inner self through
the woman's awareness of her body and the space which it occupies.
Ritual and sacred dancers would often wear a mask which would allow
their conscious mind to loosen its restrictions more easily by separating
it from the image which the body presented to the world.

If you are not confident of your ability to dance, start off by dancing
in private to recorded rhythmic music, to the rhythm of bare feet
or to the clapping of your hands. You may want to find out about
dances from other cultures and to copy some of their movements.
Wear clothes which will not restrict your movements and choose
flowing materials which will exaggerate them. Use bells, bracelets and
jewellery, especially on the arms and legs, to enhance the rhythm of
your dance.

As you start to dance, allow the rhythm to shape your steps and
thoughts. Moving to the music will gradually dissolve any sense of
embarrassment or inhibition and you will soon feel joy and pleasure
in the movement of your body. Become aware through the rhythm of
the creative energies within your body and in the world around you.
Feel yourself connected to the world through these creative energies.
Allow your feelings to express these energies through your dance into

the manifest world; dance your sexuality, your pleasure at life, your awareness, your vision, your intuition and your creativity. Allow the energy to flow from your fingers, your hair and your feet and visualize it as a radiating aura around you as you dance. Use your voice to call, to pant and to cry out as you dance, releasing the energy through your breath. In a final release, cry out and allow yourself to rest on the ground in exhaustion.

You may find that as your confidence grows, you will wish to dance with other women and you may want to enact circle or maze dances at the turning of the seasons, phases of the moon or events of life, in order to express your awareness and identification with the cycles of nature and of life.

DRUMMING

The simplest and often the oldest dances were performed to the simple rhythms set by the feet on the ground, the voice, clapping hands or by simple percussion instruments and drums. These dances can still be found in the Greek, Jewish and Native American cultures and in the dances of the whirling dervishes. The drum and the flute are the oldest types of instrument in many cultures and they held a symbolism which enhanced and augumented that of the dances which they accompanied.

The drum was a woman's instrument, its shape evocative of the encompassing circle of the earth and womb, the circle of the seasons, the moon and women themselves. The voice of the drum was the voice of the earth, the pulse of life in a mother's womb and the hidden power of life within the manifest world. To beat the drum was to call the dark mother, the Hag, the hidden source of life within the woman. The beat became the repeating rhythm of life, the moon and the menstrual cycle of womanhood. When the drumming ceased, the natural rhythms still continued.

The phallic-shaped flute was traditionally the man's instrument. The music of the flute was the voice of mortal life; it played the melody of the manifest phases of the moon which was born, waxed and waned, and died. The melody and the rhythm together expressed the nature of the divine. The melody of the individual cycle was woven into the ceaseless rhythmic cycle of the source of all life.

Like dancing, drumming can release the constraints of the intellect and awaken awareness of the inner world. The drum becomes a link with the inner world and a form of expression for the creative energies. Many cultures have their own style of drum and drumming, so choose a drum and method which you feel happy with. The simplest form of drum is a wooden hoop covered with a skin like the Irish bodhran or the instruments found in the Native American tradition and the simplest form of drumming is to hit a single beat with each stroke. Play with your drum until you find a beat which seems natural and easy to maintain and listen to the drum's voice, the reverberation which continues after it has been struck.

Feel the beat of the drum as the pulse of life, of your sexuality and creativity and the voice as the expression and form which you give to these energies. Gradually increase the strength of the beat, keeping the rhythm the same and feel the creative energies flowing through you to birth in the sound. When you feel ready, end the rhythm on a final strong beat and as you listen to the sound fade away feel the energies fade also. This type of drumming allows the energies to flow from the drummer and when accompanying a dancer, blends the energies of both drummer and dancer.

THE VOICE

Like the drum, the voice is also a way of giving form to the creative energies through sound. In modern society where people live close to each other, it is unusual for people to use their voices to maximum volume. As children, we are told not to yell or shriek and are taught that the only expressions of the voice which are acceptable to society are those which are channelled through the constraints of language and song. The idea of voice as a form of wordless expression, however, can often be found in descriptive imagery; a person shrieks with delight, laughs with happiness, cries with pleasure, wails in grief, screeches in anger and screams in pain or fear. Many of these expressions are often now viewed by society as a lack of individual control. By breaking social conditioning and expressing her emotions through the full force of her voice, a woman is able to release her creative energies, although this method may not be appropriate for every woman depending on her individual circumstances.

To try expressing the energies through your voice, you need to sit or stand comfortably with a straight back. Take in a deep breath by first of all pushing your diaphragm out and filling the base of your lungs, then expanding your chest to fill the middle of your lungs and finally filling the top of your lungs and airways with as much air as you can comfortably manage. This procedure and the release of the air may need to be practised to ensure that the action becomes smooth and automatic. Release the air in an 'ah' or 'lah' sound, by first contracting your chest and then pulling in your stomach. Keep the sound going until all the air is expelled.

Having mastered this technique, concentrate on your mouth and the force with which you expel the air. As you release the air, allow your mouth to gradually widen as far as comfortable and you will notice a strengthening of the sound. Gradually increase the force with which you release the air, allowing the sound to rise and ending with a loud cry. Experiment with different sounds; try single vowels at a constant pitch, mix them together in a rising scale or allow them to increase in strength and then fade. As you release the sound, be aware of releasing your creative energies and your sexuality, experiences and emotions through your body and feel them spiralling out of your mouth. Fit the sound you make to your feelings and for a short while forget that the neighbours think they have a banshee living next door!

Drumming, dancing and the voice can all be used together as an expression of the creative energies; the dancer and the drummer can use their voices and mix and weave their sounds, movements and rhythms together.

SEX

Sex and eroticism are the most obvious expressions of the creative energies through the body and are a powerful force in the generation of art. Sexuality offers the ability to create and to shape life. The act of sex awakens a woman's creative energies and increases her creativity and inspirational abilities or forms the body of a child around the essence of life which she carries.

In the past, a woman's sexuality was revered. All women, like the divine, had the ability to create new life and to shape the manifest world and the act of sex was seen as an experience with a strong spiritual content, beyond simple sexual gratification. Sex was a prayer, a meditation and a celebration of life and the divine. Women in the Babylonian and Sumerian cultures would offer their acts of sex at the temples as a form of worship and service to their goddess and a woman was expected to offer this form of worship at least once in her life.

The act of sex was also seen as an act of empowerment for both men and women. In many cultures, a man could only become a king if he married and mated with the representative of the Sovereignty of the land. Through this act of sex he became empowered to be king, being given the authority, responsibility, wisdom and inspiration of the goddess of the land. In return, the king, through the act of sex, awoke the creative energies within his partner and in the land, bringing fertility and fruitfulness to them both. If the king became unable to awaken these energies through age, illness, disability or neglect, the goddess's representative would turn elsewhere for her mate, her awakener.

This imagery is a common theme in folklore and is perhaps best known in the story of King Arthur, when Queen Guinevere, the representative of Sovereignty, is neglected by Arthur and turns instead to Lancelot as her lover. The direct effect of this act is that Arthur loses his power and authority over the knights and his people; gradually his knights become scattered across the country in search of the Holy Grail and the high ideals of Camelot and the Round Table are destroyed. The image of the wounded king and the subsequent devastation of the land is also found in the Grail legends in the story of the Fisher King.

Sexual intercourse links the human to the land, the man to the woman and the woman to her creative energies and thus she becomes the source of inspiration and empowerment for her partner. In history and legend, a woman has often been the source of vision, muse, enthusiasm, challenge, energy, strength and inspiration for a man, acting as a catalyst in his life, and goddesses were portrayed as giving guidance, direction and meaning to the lives of their chosen heroes.

In both ancient Greece and India, educated women who were skilled in the arts of sex were given a higher status in the courts than ordinary women. These women were valued for their ability in music and poetry and in their perception in discussions of philosophy and warfare. Their interaction with men in the sexual act brought them pleasure and the arousal of their energies and offered the men pleasure and vision. These women brought to men the art of sex, the true value of the act itself.

In the western world, the act of sex and its social acknowledgement have suffered greatly through the doctrines of the Christian Church. The idea of the body, sex and sexuality as expressions of the divine, of worship and spirituality can be difficult for even the most openminded modern person to understand. For so long, sex and sexuality have been regarded as drawing people away from the divine and women's sexuality in particular was seen as the original temptation which led mankind away from God.

In medieval Christianity the wonder, beauty and divinity of the act of sex was lost to society and as society turned away from sex, the body and nature in the search for the divine, it in effect turned away from the divine in the powers of creation. The woman's sexual role became one of submission to her husband's needs and a means by which she might bear his children. For a woman to enjoy sex, to ask for it or to gain pleasure and energy from it was seen as allowing her evil nature to surface and lost her any respect she might have had from men or society. The concept of sex became firmly linked to male gratification and the production of children and any eroticism was regarded as pornography. Even in the more 'enlightened' and 'sexually aware' modern world, the concept of sex as a spiritual expression is either unthinkable or viewed as perversion. To the modern world sex is still seen as a dirty, shameful, depraved act if it occurs outside the tightly structured, socially acceptable restrictions and strictures and, like menstruation, aspects of it are regarded as evil or, at worst, lost completely to society.

With the awakening and flow of sexual energies come inspiration, ideas, realization and the capacity to create. If you are sexually active, become aware of your creative energies through touch, movement, loving and caring whilst you are making love. Become aware of both the physical world and the world of feelings and realize that your lovemaking exists in both. Be aware of your womb and its link to the sensations of your body. Allow yourself the freedom from inhibitions to express your energies through your body and its interaction with another body. Be wild, be gentle, be passive, be caring, be animal and untamed, be graceful and poised! Feel yourself weaving your enchantment in a web which, depending on the phase of your cycle, may be the enclosing and containing web of your love, the enchantment which takes and transforms, the darkness of the inner world in the outer world or the garment of light and renewal.

Sexual energies can be released from the body in orgasm or directed through the hands or the voice. To release the energy through the hands and voice, stretch your arms above you and shout or scream your energy, feel it flowing through your voice and through your arms and out of your hands. By directing the energy to encompass yourself and your lover, you create a loving bond between the two of you on a deeper, inner level.

A woman can, if she wishes, use a man and take all of the energy he has to give. The image of the female vampire is one extreme example of a sexual woman taking all of the energies from a man to give herself life and pleasure. The female vampire reflects the Enchantress phase in the menstrual cycle, but in the cycle she is normally balanced by the other phases. It is not wrong to take when in the Enchantress phase, but this must be balanced by an awareness of giving in one of the other phases. To continually take from a relationship without giving something in return is to destroy that relationship. Treat your partner with respect, generosity and love. To love and care for someone, whether sexually, physically, emotionally or spiritually, is to express the creative energies.

Your sexuality will change with your monthly phases, so allow yourself to experience the full range of different qualities. If you do not normally make love whilst bleeding, try it. As your awareness of your different phases of sexuality grows, your partner too will become more aware of them and react differently to them. This brings variety into the relationship, but it also brings a living acceptance of the cyclic nature of a woman.

If you are not in a sexual relationship, the sexual energies may still be released through orgasm or they can be released in the other creative expressions considered. Sexual frustration, whether through restriction, self-denial or lack of opportunity, can be turned into creative flow.

Expression through the Environment

THE HOME

The sensuality of a woman bridges the distinction between her sense of self and the world around her. The environment in which she lives becomes an extension of her sense of self. This is the art of the homemaker. The creation of the feelings of comfort, security, belonging and love through the use of objects, colours, furnishings and patterns are all reflections of a woman's inner awareness. The homemaker creates a space as an outside 'body' or 'womb' in which to care for her children and her partner, family and friends. To enter a woman's home is to enter part of her inner world and this may explain why some women feel that burglary in the home can be akin to rape; the violation of the home feels like a violation of the extended body. For men, the home may be purely functional, but for a woman the home becomes part of her self.

Take note of your own home or living environment and notice how you express yourself within it. What are your feelings about the colours, the patterns, the furniture and decorations? Did you use your feelings as a guide to decorating? Are you confident about how your environment should look and what is necessary for you to feel happy in it? If you feel unhappy about something, think about changing it, try and find out what would feel right and would express your sense of self. In a family home, it can be difficult to gain this sense of self within the environment; if you are a mother, be aware that the *whole* house is the extension of your self in which you hold the environments of your children and partner. If you are in a sharing environment with others, then your own room or your sleeping area is the extension of your self. The old tradition of the son bringing home his new bride to live in the family home implied that the mother of the family, as represented by the home, accepted the new wife and allowed her to become contained within her extended 'body/womb'.

Within her living environment, a woman uses her creative energies not only in the home's outward appearance but also in its organization, management routines and traditions. She creates a sense of family through relationships, providing order, structure, security and sustenance. Cleaning the house, cooking meals, washing laundry are all expressions of women's creative energies. If a woman's environment includes a garden, that garden may reflect the link between herself and the land. Nature becomes available to the woman and she to nature, and she may choose to express this interaction by growing herbs, flowers, fruit and vegetables. The use of homegrown food and herbs for cooking and herbal remedies can reflect the link between the woman and the land in her everyday life.

LANDSCAPE ART

The environment and the sense of personal space for a woman need not be limited to the home, but can also include the land around her. Standing on a hill, viewing the vastness of the sky and the earth should not make you feel small and insignificant, but rather kindle a sense of belonging, a feeling of being a part of the whole.

Decorating the landscape as an expression of the creative energies is like decorating the home or the body; it acknowledges the space around a woman as part of that woman and reflects her own awareness of this fact. The sky and the earth become part of a woman's body, that space in which she lives. By performing art on the landscape, a woman expresses her awareness of the integration of the land and its creative energies with her sense of self and her own creative energies.

Landscape art can encompass many things. It may involve sculpture, painting, music, dance, earthwork or any activity performed outside and carried out with an awareness of the land. It may simply involve the use of decorative plants and flowers in your own garden or windowbox, or you may wish to be more ambitious and work in more public places – but be aware of the possible impact this may have on other people and on the land itself.

Use the nature around you as a medium and a source of inspiration. Tie ribbons to trees, decorate springs and wells with flowers, use stones and branches to make structures, circles and spirals and carve dead wood into interesting shapes which you can leave in place in the countryside. Create your expression in your garden, in woodlands, in fields, by rivers, on the beach, on hill tops and in caves. Look at rocks and trees for images of the female body and use non-toxic natural materials which will weather, disperse or break down to enhance or bring out the shape. Use paints made from coloured earths, ground spices mixed with water, coloured sands or natural chalk. Sand can be poured onto the earth to make pictures similar to the sand paintings of the Native American Indians and the sand mandalas of the Tibetan

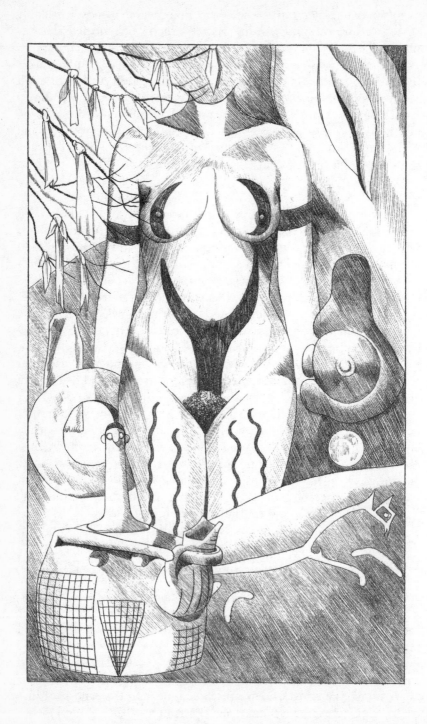

Buddhists. Even the offering of a stone at a site which you feel has special meaning for you can symbolize your presence as an expression of awareness and therefore art.

Art forms in the landscape may be large or small. They may involve only yourself or other likeminded women and may be permanent or transient. Your expressions may be altered with the moon or the season or may become a place in which to dance and feel the closeness of nature and the divine. Like the ancient stone circles, your own landscape features can be built over years of activity and observations or they may be made quickly in the creativity of the moment. They may be maintained over a long period or allowed to decay and weather, leaving the landscape as though they had never been. This emphasizes the process rather than the product. Allowing the art form to decay can be viewed in the same way as singing a note; it is first given form and then allowed to fade and die. Both the art form and the note are of the moment; neither can be recreated exactly the same and the death of the form is as powerful as its birth. The process of creation of the form is therefore also one of destruction, reflecting the cycle of life and of women.

With restrictions on ownership and laws on ecology and preserving the environment, it is important to make sure that any permanent landscape art is done with permission and that any temporary art does not damage the environment or introduce objects which, if left behind, will become litter.

Expression through the Mind

INSPIRATION AND IMAGINATION

Ideas, thoughts, imagination and intuition are all creations of the mind, which may be given form in language and writing. Inspired writing puts into words the experiences and insights of the author, often enabling her to leap mentally in awareness and inspiration. The form which the writing takes depends on the writer. The words may appear as poetry or prose, or as a descriptive passage, a story, a play or a joke.

Most people receive or write a love letter or poem at some time in their lives. These words are an expression of the writer's inner awareness and feelings. To the reader, the grammar or rhyme does not matter; the letter or poem is treasured for the process through which the writer gives form to his or her feelings, rather than the final form itself. Use your own experiences, awareness and feelings as a source of inspiration for writing. Express your feelings of energy in the words which you write. Your writing becomes a reflection of your personal development and your inner awareness.

To be creative is not just to produce physically, but also to produce mental awareness. To look at the world creatively is to create. Looking at a painting, reading a story or listening to music can therefore be seen as equally creative as actually painting the picture, writing the story or playing the instrument. You express your awareness of the world around you in the creation of thoughts and feelings. Use your creativity to make pathways through chaos, find solutions to problems, forge relationships through communication and love, discover humour and laughter, enhance knowledge and teaching, recognize beauty and insight and develop empathy and understanding.

DIVINATION AND SYMBOLIC ACTION

The modern world regards intuition, imagination and emotion as secondary to the intellect and reason, and therefore the concept of magic and ritual is derided by the scientific and intellectual community.

The art of divination uses intuition and imagination to find and make patterns. The patterns of life are all around you, but the process of divination gives us a form and structure in which the mind is able to recognize them. In using a system of divination, a woman uses her creative energies to see these patterns and to interpret their meaning.

To learn a system of divination, a woman needs to create a means of communication between her conscious mind and her inner self. This bridge may be formed by the images on a set of Tarot cards, the shapes in a system of runes or magical symbols, or the pictures formed by tea leaves. Learning the corresponding meanings is more than just an intellectual process and many systems of divination require the use of meditation, visualization and storytelling to allow each reader to find their own meanings for the images or symbols.

Having established a means of communication, the reader of the cards or symbols needs to develop the ability to quieten the rush of everyday thoughts, to become alert to the inner expression. At first, the readings may be very intellectual, using set 'rules' to fit meanings onto positions or combinations, but with practice the process becomes more intuitive, with the reader interpreting meanings from her own feelings and inner images.

If you have not tried divination before, there are many books, card decks and complete divinatory systems available which offer teaching and guidance. Some people are frightened by the concept of divination, usually through misunderstanding or lack of knowledge.

Divination is an art; it is the natural expression of the creative energies and for women in particular it provides a bridge between their awareness of the inner world and the mundane world. As you learn a system of divination and practise it, make a note on your Moon Dials of those times when you are drawn towards using it and when you find it easiest to interpret the patterns.

It is not necessary to buy an expensive deck of cards or set of runes to practise divination – you can make your own system of images and correspondences. Early divination and augury was often based on observation of the patterns of bird flight or the way in which a bundle of sticks or bones fell onto the floor. Published systems are, however, useful in guiding you by means of a structure which has already been worked out and found to be effective by someone with experience in this field, and should provide a good starting point for understanding the common methods of interpretation. It is easier still to learn a system of divination from someone who is already using it, because in this way you are able to pick up the feelings which that person associates with the images and patterns by the way they express them to you in teaching.

The art of magic can be viewed as an interaction between the tangible and the intangible worlds, awakening the creative energies through the imagination and releasing them through physical expression directed by thought and visualization. In the past, a woman would stitch her love and protection into a cloak or scabbard for her husband, weave and knot spells into ropes and threads, write a curse for bad luck for an enemy or rival or use her skills to create charms and talismans. She would knead good health and well-being into the bread she baked for her family and focus her energies on her own fertility and that of the land at full moon dances.

A symbolic action is one which expresses an inner experience of life, whether this experience manifests as a desire to direct the energies to cause an effect or as an awakening of awareness and insight. The act of lighting a candle may serve to focus the creative energies in a prayer or it may express the awareness of the divine in the person who lights it. These symbolic actions can be as simple as the 'Cleansing' exercise described on page 84 or may be much more formal and complex, depending on the preferences and needs of the individual. Wearing different colours and clothes during your phases is a symbolic act, as it expresses your inner experience. Wearing a symbol of bleeding at menstruation implies that you are taking on the powers of menstruation.

You may wish to try to direct your creative energies with purpose and intent. As you release the energies, send them out to someone in healing; as you cook the evening meal, focus your energies into the preparation to bring health and well-being. When you use your voice, project your love and caring and when you make love weave your energies into the forging of a relationship or the creation of a child.

You may wish to bring some form of symbolic action into your own life in order to acknowledge your menstrual cycle, the cycle of your life and the cycle of the earth and moon. The creation and maintenance of your Moon Dial can be made into a symbolic action, for example by using two bowls and some stones, beads or berries. You will need as many stones as the number of days in your cycle, plus a few extra if you have an irregular cycle. Decorate the stones or choose coloured beads to represent each phase of your cycle and place them all into one bowl. Each day, remove the appropriate stone and place it in the other bowl.

The idea of using a symbolic act to express your cycle and the cycle of the seasons can be taken further by performing it within the landscape. Mark a circle somewhere outside but private, perhaps in your garden, on a beach or in a wood. This can be done using stones, leaves, shells or branches to outline or by scoring the ground with a stick or chalk. Use this circle as an expression of your body, your menstrual cycle, the moon's phases, the seasons, your energies, sexuality, creativity and spirituality, or as a site to dance, to sing, to make love. Through your actions the circle becomes sacred, an acknowledgement of the divine energies and rhythms of life within you and within nature. The creation of the circle is a symbolic act and every action within the circle becomes itself part of the symbol.

Grounding

It is not always possible to release the energies in a constructive manner due to a lack of time, opportunity, materials, equipment, space, etc. If the energies are allowed to build without release, however, the resulting tension and frustration can become destructive to the woman and to others through her interaction with them. The image of the Destroyer has a very positive place within the menstrual cycle but it should reflect controlled destruction with a purpose rather than the wanton destructiveness which can arise from restriction.

Frustration caused by the feeling that the body is singing with energy which has no outlet for release can cause compulsive, erratic and self-destructive behaviour. It is therefore vitally important to have a quick and easy method of release. This 'grounding' of the energies can be achieved in several ways and uses the interaction of the woman's body and her environment to release the energies safely and harmlessly and allow her to regain equilibrium.

Grounding can take place through exercise, dance, voice or sex. In any physical exercise, the energies are quickly released through the exertions of the body. Try something dynamic which involves the whole body, such as swimming, aerobics, jogging or cycling. If you do not have the time for these forms of exertion, simply run for a little way. In adult life, unlike in childhood, there is little opportunity to run just for the pleasure of life and the expression of this pleasure. As you run be aware of the sky above you and the earth against your feet and feel the energy of your body flowing through movement into the world until you are exhausted. Even the chase for a bus can become a release if it is carried out with awareness of the flow of the energies.

Using the voice in directed sound can release the tension, frustration and energy and is often the reason why premenstrual women snap or shout. If the release of the energy through the voice is achieved in a deliberate and premeditated way through controlled sound, then the unpleasantness and repercussions of yelling or snapping may often be avoided.

The creative energies can also be released in a gentler manner. Place your hands flat on the ground and visualize energy washing down your arms, through your hands and safely into the earth. Water may also be used to carry the energy away, either by placing your hands under a running tap or by standing under a shower. Feel the water washing away the energy and carrying it safely to earth.

Creative Block

At some times in a woman's cycle she may feel uncreative and disconnected from the energies which inspire her. This disconnection can feel like a blockage lying between the woman's conscious mind and the inner world, spiritual aspects of her life. She may feel alone, no longer united with the world around her and restricted to her conscious mind as her only sense of self.

To rebuild her link between her mind and her creative energies, a woman needs to become once again more aware of her body and of her true nature. The suggestions in the previous section for awakening the creative energies and making the Moon Dials may be used to re-establish a woman's rhythm and the awareness of her body and energies in her mind. Nature itself is a great healer and restorer of the creative link and a journey away from the everyday environment into the countryside can sometimes be enough in itself to release the block.

Finally, a woman may recognize her monthly pattern of energies on an intellectual level, but she needs to actively feel and experience that pattern for it to have any meaning for her. Her intellectual expectations of the energies may not match her actual experience. The awareness of the feelings and experiences of the body and its cycle are the basis of a woman's cyclic nature, and her intellect should interpret these feelings, not dictate them.

In the modern world, with all its pressures and demands, it is difficult to live in a manner true to the female cyclic nature and to maintain a continuous inner link with the creative energies. Each month, you may find yourself maintaining this awareness for part of the time and for the rest being blocked by the pressures of ordinary life. The block can be removed and the inner awareness reawoken, however, when you recognize the existence of the block within yourself and identify the reason for its occurrence.

The art of women is the expression of their own experiences and awareness of life; it is the way in which they act, react, speak, think and feel. The modern concept of art can be stale and overformal in its expression when compared to the ever-changing, all-encompassing women's art. Recognition of the validity of all forms of women's expression in society is important if society itself is to change its attitude towards the female nature. These expressions must include those which have been neglected, forbidden or destroyed in society, but which still exist in the needs of the nature of women. They include the arts of divination, oracle, ritual, magic, ecstatic dance and women's spirituality and sexuality.

The world in which most women live is male orientated and as women's expressions reflect their inter-reaction with the world in which they live, these expressions reflect that male orientation. To break away from this male influence, a woman needs to look within and find her own true nature, unspecified by society, and to express her interaction with outside life through that true nature.

SIX

The Spiralling Moon

WOMEN'S TRADITION

Women's artwork, crafts, music, poetry and drama not only act as an expression and release of the creative energies but also provide a medium for the teaching and guidance of other women. Through the expression of their own energies and nature, women create images, symbols, concepts and archetypes which can awaken understanding and insight in others.

In the past, women's art and archetypes provided a means of guidance which helped women to understand their nature and their interaction with the cycles of life and the land. Pictures and decorations offered concepts in a visual and symbolic form, whilst stories and songs allowed the concepts to be experienced through the imagination of the listener. These ideas were offered to women not in an intellectual form but in a form which would be felt and experienced. Archetypal images grew from the experience and feelings of women and so these images would awaken those same experiences and feelings within other women who came to identify with them. As all aspects of the feminine were accepted and revered, the images, archetypes and mythology reflected this.

Stories and legends offered knowledge of the nature of women. They taught the cyclic rhythm of women's energies and their link with the land and the divine. They also taught understanding of the relationships between mother and child and between woman and man, and of the turning points in life such as birth, the first menstruation, the end of menstruation, death and rebirth. The stories of Snow White and Sleeping Beauty, for example, taught about the change from child to woman, the awakening of menstruation and the relationship between child and father and child and lover. The story of Persephone and Demeter taught about the relationship between mother and daughter, the cycles of woman and the land and life and death; and the story of Eve taught the powers of menstruation and the creative energies and the relationship between those powers and men.

By identifying with the image, each woman was able to awaken in herself the energies expressed by the archetype. By worshipping an archetype in the form of a goddess, women expressed their awareness, or their need for awareness, of that aspect of the divine feminine within themselves. Although a statue or image of a goddess would be physically separate from the woman, the female worshipper would not feel that separateness but would identify closely and directly with the image. Many of the ancient poems and invocations to the goddess which have survived from ancient Egypt and Assyria are written using the form 'I am . . .'. The woman who spoke those words identified with the divine nature within herself; she spoke as the goddess.

The destruction of these feminine images, teachings and religions which constituted the basis of a woman's tradition left women struggling in a society which offered few images of the feminine for guidance; those which were present reflected the expectations and perceptions of the male-orientated society. Christianity offered two main archetypes for women; the 'evil' Eve who disobeyed God and who through her sexuality brought death and evil into the world and the 'good' Virgin Mary who obeyed God and through the transcendence of her sexuality brought the hope of life into the world. The female saints of the Church were those who had led 'pure' lives and had done God's bidding, whilst those women who listened to their sexuality and true nature were condemned to eternal damnation. The teachings associated with these images were of the subjugation of the female nature by man or God.

The image of the Virgin Mary gradually grew in importance in the Christian religion, often taking over many of the beliefs and titles of earlier goddesses. Mary could not, however, fulfil all aspects of the feminine. The Virgin Mary was a symbol of purity; she was portrayed as a *woman* who was *physically* a virgin before, during and after the birth of her child. With the underlying belief that the first sexual act, whether with a man or snake, brought menstruation, the Virgin Mary could not be seen as a menstrual woman. The image of the Virgin Mary is one of a being beyond all other women, existing in a state which none can emulate, a woman whose role defies nature and who is truly unattainable, totally unlike the earlier goddess forms who *were* nature and therefore approachable by all women.

Modern female images have been influenced by the Christian doctrine and the expectations of men. They are found in advertising, newspapers, television programmes, films and books. Although the view of women is slowly changing, the images used of women and their roles are still restricted and channelled. Women are frequently portrayed as sexual and desirable but therefore not 'respectable' or as respectable but non-sexual. Old women are often viewed as non-sexual and undesirable, with little intellect or worth to society. Wives are portrayed as the keepers of the family and as playing a secondary role to men or they are seen as independent, shrewish, sharp-tongued nags. Women in career positions appear as selfish, singleminded and aggressive and women in male-dominated careers are often seen as unfeminine and less sexual.

The most obvious sign that some of these images are changing are the roles and characters found in commercials targeted specifically at women. These images, though, lack the completeness and the inner experience which is felt with true archetypal images. For modern women to understand their nature and how they can live in harmony with it and the modern world, there needs to be a reinstatement of the archetypes demonstrating all the different and complementary aspects of a woman's nature. Without these archetypes, the modern woman struggles to understand and accept her nature without the appropriate teaching and guidance to help her. The menstrual woman is cyclic, but she is expected to be constant and linear; she feels a part of the world around her but is told she is separate; her eroticism feels creative and spiritual but she is told that it is pornography or evil; she feels the cycling of life, but is told there is no cycle. It is little surprise that women have problems with modern society and are looking to redefine their roles within it and expectations of it.

REINSTATING THE MISSING FEMALE ARCHETYPES

The modern woman can use female images from cultures other than her own and from the past in order to reawaken the missing aspects of the feminine in modern society. Archetypes and images of the divine feminine can be found in mythology, folk stories and legends and although these stories reflect the societies in which they were originally told, the guidance offered is based on the understanding of the feminine even if it has become distorted over the years. Many of the goddesses and women featured in mythology and folklore can be placed on the Moon Dial as archetypes of the different phases. Some may also be placed in several phases, indicating that they were once recognized as representing the whole of the cycle.

The Moon Dial in Figure 9 suggests some positions for a number of

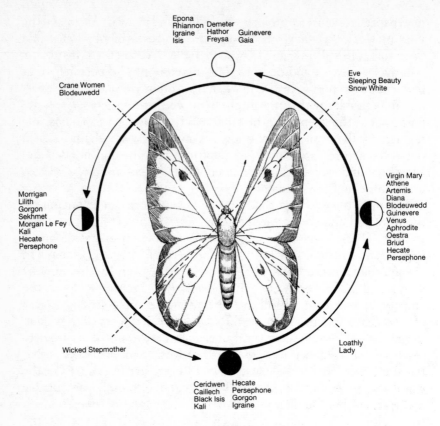

Epona
Rhiannon   Demeter
Igraine   Hathor   Guinevere
Isis   Freysa   Gaia

Eve
Sleeping Beauty
Snow White

Crane Women
Blodeuwedd

Virgin Mary
Athene
Artemis
Diana
Blodeuwedd
Guinevere
Venus
Aphrodite
Oestra
Briud
Hecate
Persephone

Morrigan
Lilith
Gorgon
Sekhmet
Morgan Le Fey
Kali
Hecate
Persephone

Wicked Stepmother

Loathly
Lady

Ceridwen   Hecate
Caillech   Persephone
Black Isis   Gorgon
Kali   Igraine

Figure 9.   Moon Dial Archetypes

goddesses and legendary women, and some of the associations attached
to the different phases of women. You may like to compare this Moon
Dial with the associations which you have developed for your own cycle
in Chapter 4. You may wish to add to the figure goddesses, women or
other associations from your own tradition or research or you may wish
to alter some of the positions.

The goddess of Sovereignty has been placed at the centre of the
dial to indicate that she can be found in folklore in all of her four
phases. The lines of transition between the phases have been allocated
to women from folklore who have already been mentioned in previous
chapters and they represent only a sample of those who could be placed
on these transition lines.

Although images and symbols from the past can be used to help
women to become aware of their true natures, it is important to adapt
or alter those older forms to become relevant for women living in the
present world or to recreate your own archetypes and stories based

on your experience of the female perception of the modern world. This lack of structured tradition is not neccessarily a bad thing, as it means that women now need to develop their own individual structures and concepts, resulting in expressions of understanding which are innovative, new, personal and constantly changing.

You could make images and archetypes based on your awareness and experiences of your own cycle or from folklore, legend or children's stories which you may have heard, and show them to other women. The archetypes need not have the form of women; they can, for example, be represented by the moon or by animals or symbols. Use crafts, painting, drawing, sculpture, writing, music, dance, ritual and drama to give form to your archetypes and to communicate your understanding and allow it to awaken in others. Celebrate any festivals in the year which you feel enhance your connection and involve your children, family and friends.

Form a group of women friends and discuss and share your experiences. Bring art into drama, music into storytelling, dance into poetry and allow women who have not tried something before to learn from a woman who has. Within the group, compile a set of images, stories, music and objects which express your experiences to become the focal point for the teaching of your children and grandchildren. Create music from the sounds and rhythms of your bodies, enhancing the bond with all women in the pattern of womanhood. Cook a meal together, expressing the archetype of nourisher and sustainer; have sessions of spinning, weaving, knitting or sewing to express the archetype of the spinner of life and creation.

GUIDING AND TEACHING YOUR CHILDREN

In the past, the traditions of the family and bloodline were held by the mother and conferred on her children. The woman taught her children the structure of the society into which they had been born and their role in it. The mother guided the new personality of her child to growth intellectually, emotionally, sexually, creatively and spiritually, through the use of stories and symbolic rites.

This role of teacher and guide has been largely taken away from the modern woman and given over to society itself. Formal teaching and schooling with set syllabuses and curricula remove the child from the mother's environment, resulting in the child's development being shaped by male-orientated society. Even within the home, the child's learning comes largely from society through television, videos, books and electronic games.

The teaching of the menstrual cycle and its meanings in the western world has become the last subject which is open to the mother to teach and which has not been taken over by society. Society ignores the menstrual cycle beyond its physical form and therefore offers no guidance to children of its experiences. Many women are conditioned to the point where they are unable to offer guidance to their own daughters and leave their education about the menstrual cycle solely to the biology class. This inability may occur because the mother has a lack of understanding of her own cycle, was traumatized by her own first menstrual experience or because she has no role model on which to base her guidance and teaching of her daughter.

The biological teaching in the science class concerning menstruation lacks any consideration of the personal experiences linked to the menstrual cycle. It does not recognize the feelings and emotions associated with the menstrual cycle and for this reason it is important for mothers to pass on to their children their own experiences and feelings relating to and extending from their own cycles. It is not only girls who need to be taught the meanings and expressions of the menstrual cycle, however, but also boys, so that they will respect womanhood and its abilities.

The mother and the grandmother need to prepare the girl for her future monthly bleeding by providing her with the language, stories and images through which to communicate understanding of the experiences of the menstrual cycle. The mother is able to give her own experiences and insights to her child as she journeys through her own monthly cycle; the grandmother, who will often be menopausal or post-menopausal, is able to offer a view from beyond the cycle.

A mother needs not only to share her experiences of her own cycle with her child, but also to set it within a framework of understanding. The mood and behaviour swings of a menstrual woman can be very daunting to a child unless they are given a stabilizing concept and this concept needs to be given to them in language and imagery which they can easily understand. For example, the love of the mother for the child may be presented simply in the image of the moon. The moon is still the moon whether you can see a crescent or the full face or when it is hidden completely in the darkness, and the mother is still the child's *loving mother*, whatever aspect she is in.

The ideas and experiences of the menstrual cycle can be introduced to the young child most easily through storytelling. Many stories from different traditions and cultures hold imagery of the menstrual cycle within their women characters, goddesses and faery queens and in their interaction with each other, the land and the moon. Use the imagery from the stories to describe yourself; tell your child that you feel like an enchantress (editing the usual 'evil') or like the young Snow White. Explain the role of the characters in the stories, perhaps by becoming that character for the child. In the case of Snow White, the Enchantress/stepmother was helping Snow White to grow up. Use stories like *The Loathly Lady* to explain that you yourself are sometimes like the old woman, but then you change once again into a young woman.

Your phases can also be expressed to your child through the seasons or with Moon Animals. You can describe yourself as feeling like summer, bright and warm and happy, or like an owl, dark and quiet and beautiful. By using stories, you are using images to which you can relate and with which the child can also identify. It is, however, important that the child understands that whatever animal, season or character you are like at the moment, your love for your child remains the same.

You may also wish to involve your child in your individual expressions of your creative energies. Cook, dance, play music, paint and make landscape pictures together. Include the child in your symbolic actions, explaining what they represent. If you are able, allow other women to interact with your child also, sharing their own stories and expressions. These women may be grandmothers, aunts, sisters or your close friends and they can offer your child another view of the menstrual cycle as well as awakening in them the idea that other women also change.

In using yourself and your experiences as a basis for teaching your children, allow them to guide you through their own questions on how much they want or are ready to know. As your daughters get older, you may wish to start going into greater detail. The story of *The Awakening* can be used for this purpose if you are unsure about creating your own story, adapting the language and imagery to suit the level of your daughter's understanding. Offer your child your own archetypal images, explaining and teaching about their meanings.

By making your daughters and sons aware of your own menstrual cycle and the daughters' future cycle, the event of the first bleeding can become one of family acceptance and will hold no fear or embarrassment.

RITES OF PASSAGE

One of the most ancient forms in which to introduce ideas and experiences was the use of the rite of passage. These symbolic or ritual events marked the transition of an individual from one phase of their lives into a new phase of awareness and perception. These rites often marked a change in status in the community, for example at puberty, marriage, at the making of a priest/priestess or a king and usually resulted in a change in the legal or social restrictions and obligations of the individual.

In the western world the concept of the rite of passage has gradually become eroded, especially that relating to puberty. Echoes of the original idea remain in the concept of 'coming of age' which is accompanied by certain legal rights and obligations, but even this landmark has lost status because of the varying ages at which the different legal restrictions on behaviour are released. Without a rite of passage, the modern child has no specific point at which they become a young adult and they may oscillate between child and adult, unsure of the expectations of their parents, society and the law.

The rite of passage for a girl needs to mark not only the change from childhood to the start of adulthood but also the start of womanhood. The physical act of a girl's first bleeding is her natural rite of passage and it is only in relatively recent times that this has been ignored. The girl's life changes in that one event from the linear nature of childhood to the cyclic nature of womanhood. A symbolic act at the time of first bleeding recognizes, emphasizes and accepts the change which has occurred in the child and becomes for that child the start of learning from her own experiences as she grows into maturity.

The change within the child cannot just be marked intellectually; she needs to *feel* that she has passed into young womanhood. This feeling can be created by a symbolic rite of passage, but it also needs to be reinforced later through the reactions and expectations of parents and other family members. The child needs to learn about the responsibilities and skills she will need for adult life but also about her own nature as a woman. In the past, the seclusion of a girl after first bleeding until maturity was intended to teach her all aspects of womanhood; the acceptance and use of the abilities and energies which arose with her different phases as well as the more mundane skills associated with being a wife and a mother.

The First Blood Rite of Passage

The female nature expresses itself through a woman's feelings and so the symbolic act of passage into womanhood will need to feel right for your daughter and reflect her own emotional, intuitive and inspirational needs. The female nature also expresses itself through the body and its sensations and through its interaction with the environment surrounding it, so it is important to set the rite in a place which creates the correct atmosphere for your daughter.

Think about an environment for your child's rite and ask yourself what colours, music, objects and movement would be most reassuring for her. What emotions do you wish her to feel and what will cause them to arise in her? Would she like to be outside or within the house? Is she shy and would therefore respond better to a rite involving just you and her? Is she imaginative or will she need objects to help her? How confident is your daughter of her body? Would she be happier nude, costumed or in ordinary clothes, still or dancing? Will she need a feeling of magic and enchantment to inspire her? What sort of interest does she have in the different aspects of the menstrual cycle and how long is her attention span? Will she need a physical expression other than her own bleeding to show that the rite has occurred? Of course, you should discuss all this with your daughter to discover her own wishes.

The rite is for your child, to awaken the idea and the experience of womanhood within her and so needs to be designed to suit her. She may start menstruation earlier or later than her friends so be prepared to allay any anxieties this may cause. Be prepared mentally with an idea of what you intend to do, so that you are ready and able to perform it whenever she begins her first bleeding. It is not absolutely necessary to perform the rite at first bleeding, but it is best not to leave it too long afterwards, as the intention is to mark the start of her progress into womanhood.

It may be that your daughter may experience some difficulties with her first bleeding, whether physically or emotionally, so be flexible in your ideas to suit her reaction. Most importantly, consider how you yourself are going to react to her bleeding, as this will inevitably affect the way she feels about her blood and future bleedings and possibly her reaction to her own future children's menstruation.

Imagery for the rite of first bleeding can be taken from various sources. Many of the stories which include menstrual and, in particular, first blood imagery involve a maiden who withdraws from the world after coming into contact with a symbol of life and menstruation. In *Snow White*, the maiden sleeps as though dead after eating the fruit of the tree of life and in *Sleeping Beauty* the maiden sleeps after her bleeding starts, brought about by the spindle of life.

This concept of passing through darkness and awakening into new life is a lunar one and lies at the heart of the menstrual cycle and rites of passage. On awakening, the maiden has become a woman and is in possession of all the gifts of womanhood. The encounter which causes the fall into darkness often involves a fruit, which represents the menstrual fruit of the tree of life. This can be symbolized in the rite by a red apple as in the story of Snow White or by a pomegranate, olives, figs or the berries of the rowan tree. (The red berries of the rowan tree or mountain ash (*Sorbus Aucuparia*) are not poisonous, but are extremely bitter when raw and only made palatable with cooking.

Animal images such as the unicorn and the butterfly may also be used in the rite. The unicorn offers a symbol of the commencement of menstruation and its associated lunar powers which is familiar and attractive to modern girls. The presence of a girl's first blood shows that she has attracted her own unicorn and that they are bonded for the length of her menstrual life. The rite could use the folklore story of the hunting of the unicorn and mix with it with the imagery of the other menstrual stories. The butterfly is also a symbol of the lunar/menstrual cycle and its life cycle can be used as an image of the change from childhood to womanhood. Here the withdrawal of first menstruation can be represented by the chrysalis stage of the butterfly's life.

One of the most powerful and complex stories containing menstrual and first blood imagery, as well as other symbolism, is the tale of the Greek goddesses Persephone and Demeter. The story not only illustrates the path of the maiden at first blood but also offers guidance to the mother for her role in her daughter's first bleeding.

The story of Persephone and Demeter begins when Demeter, the goddess of the fruits of the earth, lived with her daughter in a land which knew no winter and the two enjoyed a close and loving relationship. One day, whilst picking flowers in a field, Persephone was irresistibly drawn to a magical narcissus plant, which shone with beauty and filled the air with a wonderful scent. As Persephone reached out and touched the plant, the earth opened up and she was abducted into the darkness of the earth by the lord of the underworld and forced to become his wife.

When Hecate brought her the news of the abduction of her daughter, Demeter, in grief and pain, withdrew her fertility from the land so that it existed in a perpetual state of winter and sterility and she herself became an old woman. Moved by Demeter's entreaties, Zeus finally commanded the lord of the underworld to release Persephone, which he agreed to do. Despite initially refusing to eat or to take anything from the underworld realm, Persephone had, however, eventually been tempted into consuming a handful of pomegranate seeds. The reunion between Persephone and Demeter was joyous, but when Demeter heard that her daughter had eaten the pomegranate seeds, she realized that Persephone still belonged in part to the lord of the underworld. In eventual compromise, Demeter allowed Persephone to return to the underworld for part of the year, on the understanding that she would return to spend the rest of the time in the world above with Demeter.

The story of Persephone and Demeter can be interpreted in several different ways but the core of the story, that is, the concept of the repeating cycle, is shown in all the interpretations. In relation to the land, Demeter was the goddess of the fruits of the earth, and in particular the corn, and her daughter was the life force of the earth and of the corn seed. Persephone's descent into the underworld echoed the withdrawal of the creative energies from the earth, leaving the land, her mother, as an old woman in sterile winter. The subsequent ascent renewed the life in the earth as spring and made Persephone's mother young again. Persephone, as the corn seed, was seen to be buried in the underworld of death during the winter, to reawaken into new life in the spring. She symbolized the death and rebirth of the spirit.

The story also holds strong menstrual and first bleeding imagery. Persephone is the virgin maiden who is made to withdraw from the everyday world into the darkness of the underworld. The lord of the underworld makes her his wife, giving her her first sexual experience, and tempts her into eating the fruit from the tree of life, the pomegranate. The role of the lord of the underworld in this story is interchangeable with the role of the snake in other stories. The snake was regarded as an underworld creature which guarded the tree of life and its fruits of menstruation.

When Persephone returned to Demeter, Demeter realized that because her daughter had eaten the menstrual fruit, she no longer belonged solely to her, but also to the darkness of the underworld. Demeter eventually accepts the cyclic pattern and dual nature of her child, and allows her rhythmic descent into the darkness of menstruation. Only through her descent is Persephone able to become a woman and a mother. In some of the stories attached to Persephone, she is portrayed as returning to the world with a child as a result of her union with the lord of the underworld.

The path of Persephone to first bleeding is inevitable and breaks the mother–child link between her and Demeter. Persephone can never be a child again after eating the fruit of menstruation. The break causes Demeter great pain and she mourns the loss of her child, but although she has lost the original link between mother and child, she eventually realizes and accepts that she has gained the link of womanhood with her daughter. This link is expressed in the menstruation of Demeter, the withdrawal of her fertility from the land and her image as an old woman at the time when her daughter descends into her own menstruation.

By being allowed to descend repeatedly into the underworld, Persephone is able to release the creative gifts of womanhood into the world. As a woman descends like Persephone into the underworld of menstruation each month, she feels a sense of loss and, like Demeter, she becomes an old barren woman in the winter of her cycle. Within the underworld, she becomes renewed and young again, turning her energies outward and reawakening her fertility and dynamic energies. The menstruating woman is both Persephone and Demeter; Demeter is her body and Persephone her awareness and creative energies.

Persephone can also represent the lunar concept of new life inherent in the old. Persephone as the child of Demeter is physically part of Demeter; she is the new moon growing into light, whilst Demeter is the full moon growing into darkness. Persephone is Demeter's past and her future and Demeter is Persephone's future and her past. The cycle is endless and the goddesses are merely different aspects of the same cycle or goddess.

Although this is complex imagery for a child to understand, it can be used in a rite in order to allow the child to identify with and feel the withdrawal and return of Persephone. The symbolism may be explained through gradual teaching as the child grows into maturity. Some of the imagery of the original story may need to be adapted to suit the level of understanding of your own daughter and to avoid her being frightened. In particular, the abduction scene may be altered to one in which Persephone is irresistibly called by the beauty of the voice of the lord of the underworld.

The story of Persephone and Demeter guides the mother through her identification with Demeter. The mother needs to feel the loss of her daughter and the ensuing grief if she is to accept the change which has taken place in her child. Not only does she need to accept this change herself, but she also needs to be clearly seen by the child as accepting the change and the new bond forming between her and her daughter. In a girl's rite of passage, as well as the child *feeling* the change which has occurred in her it is necessary for the mother to *feel* it as well.

On the occasion of your daughter's first blood, try to spend extra time with her as a way of expressing this special link between you and her and as an opportunity for you to teach and for her to ask questions. Above all, it gives you an opportunity to show your love and offer support and reassurance. Try to make the whole day of the rite of passage special for your daughter; do something together which is normally considered a treat and make it a family occasion if you feel that this is appropriate.

The setting and imagery for your daughter's rite of passage will depend on her needs and awareness and on your own traditions, perception and beliefs. The following guidelines may, however, help in setting some structure to the rite. They may be included in any order.

1.   Some form of affirmation of the continuing love and support of the mother for the daughter.
2.   The symbolic death of the child and the grief of the mother, and the awakening of the young woman and the joy of the mother.
3.   Some element of teaching, which may include: the meaning of the rite and the symbols/imagery used; the gifts of womanhood; the duality of woman; her link with the moon and seasons; the need for the monthly descent to bring the creative energies into the world; the strengths and beauty which come with womanhood; and the need for the child to try to remember her dreams during the period of first blood.
4.   The welcome of the daughter into the sisterhood of all women and the moon.

You may wish to involve other women in your daughter's rite and include female relatives and friends, but be aware of how your daughter may feel about being in a group. You may also want to choose a number of women who will become active in the teaching and guidance of your daughter towards her understanding of her cycle and her energies. These women could be seen as 'faery godmothers' or 'moon mothers' bringing initiation and change into a girl's life, teaching her to value her menstruation as a gift without the need for shame, hatred or guilt. The rite may end with giving the young woman a physical symbol of her change into womanhood. You could bind her hair with red ribbons, showing the binding and weaving of the menstrual cycle and the creative energies, give her a simple girdle made from the threads of your own or a gift of an image of a unicorn, a butterfly, a moon, an apple or any symbol which would have meaning for you and for her. After the rite celebrate in some way, perhaps with a family meal. The passage into womanhood is an event of celebration, not only for your daughter but also for yourself, the child's father and any other members of the family.

THE MENSTRUAL DAUGHTER

After first bleeding, the process of guiding your daughter towards knowledge of her own cycle begins. Encourage her to start keeping a record of her feelings and dreams and help her to interpret any menstrual imagery or Moon Animals which she may encounter.

Gradually build these records into her first Moon Dial. Keep your own record of your daughter's phases, moods and expressions and use these records with her Moon Dial as a basis for guiding her understanding and helping her to cope with the demands of life and her nature. Until she herself has the awareness of her cycle and the outlets to release her energies with control, you will need to provide these for her.

Show your daughter your own Moon Dials, if you have not already done so, and allow her to see how you interpret and express your own cycle, comparing it with hers. Give her understanding when she cannot cope with the demands of her nature and body and of society, and in return you will receive her understanding. Do not, however, give her the expectation of an ideal which she has to live up to, but rather give her the understanding that in modern society, which is not woman orientated, she will oscillate between being true to her nature and true to society. Teach her that balance is not easy and that she should not attach any guilt to the fact that it is not possible to achieve a balance all the time.

Help your daughter to find releases and expressions of the energies which suit her. Involve her in your own expressions, but do not expect them to be appropriate for her. Guide her in the forming of images and symbols which express the way she feels and which she can identify with, and help her to give them form in paintings, music, Moon Dials, dance and crafts. If she has a girdle, teach her to use it as a physical form of the expression of her cycle and tell her about the symbolism of your own girdle.

Continue the role of storytelling in your daughter's teaching, but begin to show her how to use the stories as visualizations and meditations. You may wish to use some of the visualizations in this book or create your own.

Be guided by your child in how much she wishes to know, how much she wants to learn from you and how much she wants to learn on her own. As your daughter develops and matures, you may find that her physical cycle, her awareness of her phases, her interpretation and expression of her cycle may be very different from your own. You may find that she brings a new approach which you had not appreciated or that she renews your own needs to express your cycle in new and exciting ways. Remember that the energies and perception of the maiden or young woman which you once were still live in you once a month and use this phase to help you to identify with the stage your daughter is going through. As your child increases in awareness of her own cycle, she may be able to understand you better too, through her experience of her own mother phase.

The knowledge of the cyclic nature of women needs to be awoken in girls and although the interpretations will change through the generations, the basic core of the nature of women and its related energies will run true. This is the 'female tradition' which you pass on to your child; not the language, the symbols or the imagery, but rather the awareness and experience and the expression of the cyclic nature through the creative energies.

The role in passing on this tradition is not just for women who are mothers and have girl children. All women, through their expression and acceptance of the nature of the menstrual cycle and its energies, offer guidance to others. The acceptance of the ways in which other women express their spirituality, their sexuality and their creativity acknowledges and gives respect to the gifts of womanhood, regardless of their form or interpretation. The expression of this in music, drama, dance, storytelling, etc. forms a collection of images and archetypes which offer society a view of the whole of the feminine nature. The power of archetypes and menstrual images runs deeper than the intellect and once they are awoken in society, society will react to them. All women, whether young girls, wives, mothers, menopausal, post-menopausal or grandmothers, have a part in the teaching of the awareness and acceptance of womanhood to other women, as well as to children and mankind.

The Rite of Motherhood

Another rite of passage which is no longer celebrated is the loss of menstruation through pregnancy and the awakening into motherhood. Although the act of birth itself constitutes the physical aspect of the change in a woman, women are often left feeling that their experience of modern childbirth does not satisfy their inner and emotional needs.

The pregnant woman loses her monthly cyclic nature at conception and progressively attunes to the changes in her body leading towards the growth of her child and its eventual birth. Like the menopausal woman, the pregnant woman steps outside the rhythm of the menstrual cycle; but whereas the menopausal woman remains in the dark moon inner phase, the pregnant woman remains in the full moon outer phase. She holds in her body the new life growing like the increasing light of the waxing moon. Her creative energies are given form in the outer world in the physical formation of her child, in the emotional bonds between the woman and her growing child, in the formation of bonds of parenthood with her partner and in the creation of a safe and secure environment into which to bring her child. She becomes a physical bridge between the two worlds through her body, becoming a doorway between the manifest and the unmanifest.

In folklore and legend, the mother's role is often one of guidance, dedication, compassion, love, caring and understanding for her child, but she may also appear as the source of the stories themselves and as the catalyst which changes events. It is often the mother's actions, the circumstances of her becoming a mother or her death which force the hero/heroine into the events and challenges of the story. Unlike the soft, passive role sometimes seen in modern images, the mother's role in the past was generally viewed as one of strength and of forcing growth and awareness. The change from a woman into a mother gives a deep inner strength not previously experienced.

The birth of a child marks a change in a woman's perception of life, from a concentration on the importance of the freedom of the individual to the dedication and responsibility of a mother with a child. She becomes the one who nourishes and supports others, embodying the legendary images of the earth mother, the Holy Grail, the white mare of Sovereignty and the full moon. Like many ancient goddesses, she holds the titles of the Lady of Life, the Lady of Joy and Abundance, the Maker of Kings and the Open Womb. It is the lack of recognition of these images and feelings by modern society which needs to be overcome by the reintroduction of a contemporary rite of passage for the occasion of motherhood.

After childbirth women return physically to their menstrual cycle, but they also need to return to it mentally. Leaving the Mother phase after the birth, the woman withdraws into her inner darkness in the need to renew and to return to her cyclic nature. This withdrawal may be felt as depression unless the woman recognizes her need for this renewal in order for her creative energies to be brought once more into the outer world. The withdrawal should not result in any guilt or the feeling of being a bad mother, but should be accepted as the source of her future energies. Some form of rite of passage after the birth may help a woman to accept this.

A rite of passage into motherhood may be split into two parts, a preliminary symbolic act linked with the pregnancy and the awakening of the woman into motherhood with the birth of her child. The preliminary act could involve imagery associated with the woman's leaving of her menstrual rhythm to remain in her Mother phase during pregnancy and the identification of the growing life within her with the moon or the land. The main rite after the birth could involve the awakening of the woman into her role as a mother, the recognition and welcome of this new phase of her life and the coming return to her cyclic nature.

These two symbolic acts which together constitute the rite of passage recognize and provide the spiritual aspect of the processes of pregnancy and birth which are missing from modern orthodox religion and birth methods.

The Rite of Menopause

Rites of passage may also occur at other times in a woman's life; some, like marriage, are still celebrated but others are not and have left a need in women for the expression of their transition. Menopause, like first bleeding, is a dramatic change in the physical expression and mental perception of womanhood and as such needs some form of recognition.

Menopause affects women in different ways and may start with the regular menstrual rhythm becoming increasingly erratic. A woman who has been aware of her phases throughout her menstrual life is able to accept more readily the symptoms and the meaning of menopause than is a woman who has no knowledge of her true nature. To the aware woman, the erratic cycles are final gifts to be used before her rhythms eventually cease and her cyclic perception and cyclic energies are ended. Like the child, the post-menopausal woman focuses all her creative energies in one direction; but unlike the outward orientation of the child's energies, the post-menopausal woman's energies are directed inward. If the energies of a child are viewed as linear and those of the menstrual woman cyclic, then the energies of the post-menopausal woman can be considered as a point or a source.

Menstrual womanhood consists of a series of descents into the inner world at menstruation in order to renew and bring back the creative energies into the outer world. The menopausal woman descends into her inner darkness but sometimes does not return renewed to her young phase through the release of blood. Eventually, she no longer passes through the transformation at all and rests in the innerworld phase. Unlike the menstrual woman, her energies do not manifest in the material world but are instead given form in her inner world. Her perception of life is no longer cyclic, but a balance between the inner and outer worlds.

From this vantage point of constant awareness of both worlds, the post-menopausal woman is by her own nature a priestess, shaman, healer and seer. She has continuous access to the inner world dimension of life which is only accessible to the menstrual woman once a month. This awareness and insight found in older women was widely recognized in past cultures, where such women were revered as counsellors, guides and holders of tradition and as the link between the spirit or ancestral world and the community.

In the Grail legends, the ageing Igraine, mother of King Arthur, withdrew from the court into the otherworld to rule the Castle of Maidens. Although no longer active in the earthly court, she influenced and guided it from the otherworld and was seen as the holder of female tradition and the weaver of the destiny of her child. Like the post-menopausal woman, she resides in the inner world, perceiving and interacting with the outer world but with an innerworld perspective. She is not portrayed as weak, decaying and frail, but rather as strong and powerful.

As queen of the Castle of Maidens, the symbol of Igraine reflects the teaching role which a post-menopausal woman has for younger women and in particular for the newly menstrual girl. The older woman in the rite of first bleeding represents in her person the inner dimension which runs through all the phases of the menstrual cycle. Her perception is not restricted by the phase of her menstrual cycles; she is beyond them and within them all and she embodies the *whole* of the cycle. As a post-menopausal woman, she holds the experience of her menstrual past and has the ability to touch the future, and her experiences bring a confidence concerning death and the cyclic nature of life which she can pass on through teaching. She *is* the phase of menstruation and, through her retention of her menstrual energies and blood, she *is* the menstrual blood. In *Snow White* and *Sleeping Beauty* it is the old woman who brings the start of menstruation, because in these stories she represents in herself the blood of the first shedding.

The post-menopausal woman has the ability to offer the child her knowledge and experience of the inner world, the divine creative source and the spiral of lineage. She also has the ability to love and care for all others, beyond the role of nourisher and sustainer but as an initiator into spiritual awareness. Even in the very materialistic modern society, this innerworld and spiritual dimension is reflected in the large numbers of older women who make up religious and spiritual congregations. As the post-menopausal woman is an active spiritual guide and initiator, all premenopausal women are her daughters and all other post-menopausal women her sisters.

The rite of passage at menopause marks an acceptance of the death of the woman's old, cyclic perception and her awakening into the innerworld. It marks the woman's final descent into the darkness to become the queen of the underworld, the guider of souls and the dark mother. As with the rite of first bleeding, the person who is undergoing the ritual needs to feel afterwards that a change in awareness and life has occurred and so the rite will need to be tailored to the individual. The following suggested inclusions may give a structure on which the individual rite may be based.

1. The acceptance of the past and the grief at its passing.
2. The final descent into darkness and the death of the old perception.
3. The awakening to darkness as queen of the underworld or dark mother.

Whether you decide to do the rite at the commencement of menopause or at the end, the following visualization may be used as part of the rite in order to help you to accept and realize the change through which you are passing.

Exercise: The Menopause Visualization

Perform the visualization in a darkened room. Begin by lighting a candle in front of you and closing your eyes. Gently relax your body and breathe deeply.

Visualize yourself standing on the plain described in the Girdle Visualization on page 107. You watch the rising crescent moon in the east fill until it becomes the full moon in the south and then reduce in the west, setting into the darkness of the north. Watch this rhythm for a few cycles and feel the rhythm of the energies associated with the different phases flow across your body and mind. Allow your awareness of the energies to follow the descent of the waning moon into the darkness of the dark moon and remain in the darkness. See the crescent moon rise from you, fill into the full moon and return in waning crescent to you. Feel your darkness surround each light phase, giving it form; you are no longer attached to the cycle, you *are* the cycle.

Spend time within the darkness watching the moon's cycle until you are ready to return to the outer world. Open your eyes and look at the candle, feeling that you are now the darkness surrounding the flame through which its light becomes manifest.

The way in which a woman views her future without her menstrual cycle will depend on how she has spent her menstrual life. For many women, the release from their cycle ends their phase of orientation towards the needs of others and begins a phase in which they may experience their lives for themselves. A rite of passage at menopause allows a woman to accept her past, to grieve for its loss and to focus on her new perception of life. It allows the woman to feel the end of one part of her life and the beginning of a new and exciting one.

To become menopausal is sometimes viewed as a sign of decay, increasing uselessness and the first indications of death; but like the individual phases in the menstrual cycle, it is just one phase in the cycle of life which, when welcomed and accepted for itself can offer women a greater satisfaction and expression in life. In her menstrual life the post-menopausal woman has already been in each month all the phases of her own life and so the energies of the old woman and the final transformation at death need hold no fear for her.

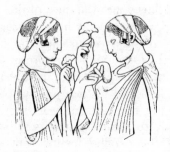

Afterword

Your understanding of and interaction with your menstrual cycle is a process of learning which will continue throughout your menstrual life. This will not result in a sudden alteration in the symptoms or the regularity of your cycle, but you will begin to accept, understand and welcome the abilities and energies which each phase brings and to balance them in your life. There will be times when the demands and commitments of modern life make it difficult for you to be fully aware of your nature as a woman. Nevertheless, you will still have the ability to reawaken the link between your mind, body and creative energies whenever you have the opportunity.

The awareness and knowledge gained through the menstrual cycle wax and wane like the moon. Insight gained through experience in one phase of the cycle can be lost in another, so that the pursuit for knowledge of the menstrual cycle becomes a continuous spiral throughout a woman's menstrual life in which she is always learning and relearning. The only constant is the here and now, the phase which you are currently experiencing and the perception and knowledge which it brings.

Red Moon began with a story offering images of the nature of women. Stories of the menstrual cycle and the gifts of womanhood were told in the past and will continue to be told in the future, forever changing in perception and interpretation and forever remaining the same. The story of women's nature has no definitive meaning, no beginning and no end, but it is one which lives in all women.

Further Reading

ADULT BOOKS

Baring, A. and Cashford, J. *The Myth of the Goddess*, **Viking** Arkana, 1991.

Durdin-Robertson, L. *The Year of the Goddess*, Aquarian, 1990.

Gadon, E. W. *The Once and Future Goddess*, Aquarian, 1990.

George, D. *Mysteries of the Dark Moon*, Harper San Francisco, 1992.

Evans, P. and Deehan, G. *The Keys to Creativity*, Grafton Books, 1988.

Harding, E. M. *Woman's Mysteries*, Rider, 1988.

Matthews, C. *Arthur and the Sovereignty of Britain*, Arkana, 1989.

Matthews, J. (ed.) *At the Table of the Grail*, Arkana, 1987.

Shuttle, P. and Redgrove, P. *The Wise Wound*, Paladin/Grafton Books, 1989.

CHILDREN'S BOOKS

Poole, J. *Snow White*, Hutchinson Children's Books, 1991.

Index